RAZOR FREE

*The Mind-Body Method
of Natural Hair Removal*

SHLOMIT KARNI

Producer & International Distributor
eBookPro Publishing
www.ebook-pro.com

RAZOR FREE
Shlomit Karni

Copyright © 2023 Shlomit Karni

All rights reserved; No parts of this book may be reproduced or transmitted in any form or by any means, electronic or mechanical, including photocopying, recording, taping, or by any information retrieval system, without the permission, in writing, of the author.

Translation from Hebrew by Noelle Canin

Contact: ehair@gmail.com

Copyright © 2020 Adi Terem and Moran Bardea, Scene 1

The quoted section or any parts of it may not be reproduced or transmitted in any form or by any means, electronic or mechanical, including photocopying, recording, taping, or by any information retrieval system, without the permission, in writing, of Adi Terem and Moran Bardea.

Contact: contact@muarim.com

ISBN 9798387006616

For my Family

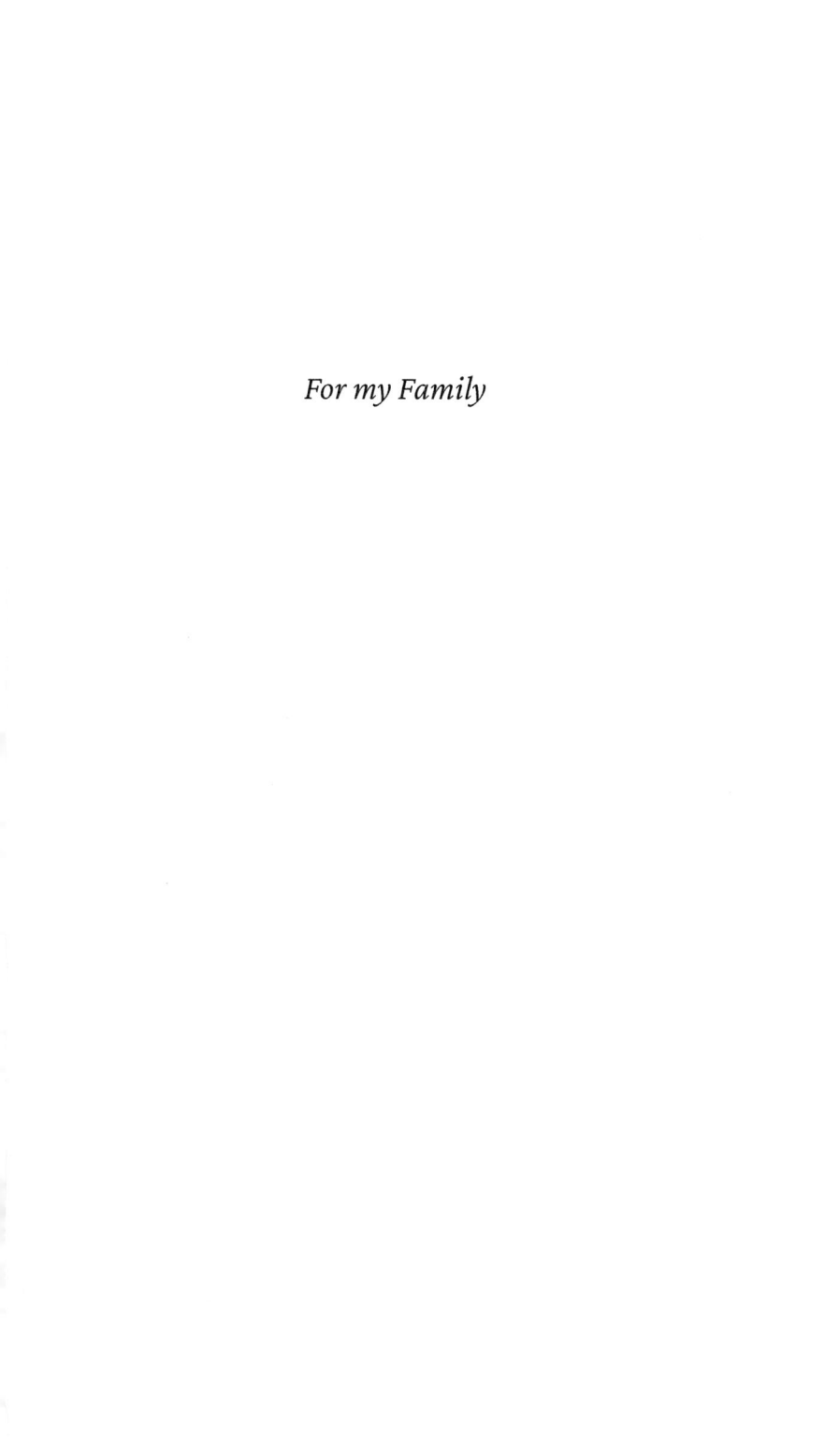

*"Everyone knew it was impossible,
until a fool who didn't know
came along and did it."*

Albert Einstein

CONTENTS

The Consciousness of a Housewife	11
Knowledge Sets Us Free	19
"The God Particle"	23
Theory	29
The Presentation	33
The Guide	37
A Pink Mustache	41
External Research	47
An Experiment that Went Wrong	53
A Little Girl	55
Routine	63
Celebrity Hair	65
Help	71
The Mouse	77
Alone?	83
Schrödinger's Cat	89
Joy that Works	97
Once too Often	101
Children Make You Grow	105

Difficult Hair	117
Enlightened Ltd	119
A Story	133
First Haircut	137
Additional Aspects of Energy Hair Experiments	143
Natural Straightening	145
Hair Garden	149
A Head of Grass	153
Balance	155
The End of the Experiment	159
Doubts	163
What Does One Do with a Theory	167
How to Remove Hair Through Energy	177

A loud scream came out of my mouth. I was shocked by the force of the pain.

My sister looked at me with disappointment.

"I'm not a doll," I grumbled.

My sister, ten years older than me, pulled one hair after another from my mustache. She was using silver metal tweezers and it hurt so much that I couldn't sit still and kept pushing her hand away.

She very quickly lost patience. "One must suffer to be beautiful," she scolded, giving me a long meaningful look through her doll-like bangs and puffy curls. Her eyes, focused on me with deadly seriousness, convinced me. She sounded as if she knew what she was talking about. I believed her. I realized I had no choice but to shut my mouth and behave like a mature woman. My innocence shattered, I realized I was doomed to go through my first ritual in a world of maturity and pain where women had to suffer for their beauty.

Resigned, I found the strength to deal with the pain and get the process over with as quickly as possible. I bit my lips, closed my eyes, and refrained from making a sound. Every now and then I glanced in the little mirror to check on the progress until, at last, my upper lip was smooth. Thanking my sister, I rushed out of the room. Descending five steps, I turned right towards the open front door that let in a scatter of sun rays. I ran out to the neighbor's house. My girlfriend, who was the same age as me, opened the door. She looked at me, saying at once, "you look different; it's as if your face is lit up."

I smiled with satisfaction, feeling that every minute of suffering had been worth it.

Twenty-Five Years Later

The Consciousness of a Housewife

It was late in the evening. Raindrops slid down the kitchen window. I switched on the kettle.

Going into the living room, I sat down on the brown fabric sofa next to my husband Gabriel who was looking thoughtful. He was twirling a green plastic Fidget Spinner with a swift and mesmerizing motion. Out of nowhere, I heard myself say: "I've been talking to the hair on my body once a month for a year now and I find that it works."

"What works?" He was focused on the spinner.

I leaned towards him and said: "With two facts, I can convince you that I can permanently get rid of body hair just by talking to it." He wasn't looking at me but I knew he was listening, so I went on: "The first fact is that plants are aware. When they are spoken to negatively, they dry and wither."

"I know," he said.

"The second fact is that each cell in our bodies is aware." I stopped, hoping he'd continue the line of thought, but Gabriel was silent. I went on, "since it's possible to talk to plants and cause them to dry and wither, it's also possible to talk to body hair and make it gradually dry up and stop growing."

I waved my hands to indicate the irrefutability of the argument I'd expressed.

"Okay," he responded, glancing briefly at me.

I hadn't expected an enthusiastic response.

"It's easy to understand because they have a deeply meaningful common denominator: consciousness," I emphasized again.

I was trying to lead him neatly toward insights I'd had over the years, and maybe I was trying to get a more empathic response.

"Did you know the spinner was invented for problems related to ADHD?" He spun the spinner once more.

"Don't you get it? During the seventies, an incredible book came out called *The Secret Life of Plants*[1], revealing that plants are sentient and absorb information from their surroundings. The book received terrible reviews from scientists at the time but, despite this, many people believed that God can create plants that have awareness. Maybe they wanted to believe in the magic that exists in the world. Rational scientists wouldn't give their seal of approval to truth without evidence of scientific research. The good news is that today, science completely concurs with the fact that plants respond to people's emotions and have a life of their own. That's just how it is; science and research are slower than human intuition."

Looking skeptical, Gabriel leaned back against the sofa. "In a nutshell," I hurried to conclude before he lost interest, "when the book about plants came out, housewives fell in

---

1. *The Secret Life of Plants* by Peter Tompkins and Christopher Bird, translated into Hebrew by Naomi Carmel, Kinneret Zmora-Bitan Publishing House, 1978.

love with the idea and talked to their house plants. So I'm just a different version of the same thing: a housewife who talks to her body hair."

"Housewives seem to have a lot of time on their hands," observed my man.

"Is that all you have to say?" I asked.

"Weren't you going to make tea?"

"It's so satisfying to see how hair responds to a few sporadic sentences; it's better than watching a science fiction movie at the cinema, and so much better than just having painful and corny old laser treatments. I was the main researcher in my 'lab' and the first to see the results of the experiment on my body: how the hair became lighter, finer, and weaker, and how the energy of the hair changed. It's exciting to see how hair does what I tell it to do. It's an incredible feeling to know that I'm no longer stuck in the body I was given, nor a victim of hair growing on me without my having a say in what I want."

Gabriel nodded and gazed at me for a long time. I wondered if he understood. I shrugged. "It's a leap for humanity, from the level of doing - to being."

"So what's next?" He asked.

"The world must be told," I tried not to sound too dramatic and jumped off the sofa to go to the kitchen.

"Okay," his response was laconic.

"Michio Kaku, Professor of Theoretical Physics, said, "even a thermostat has consciousness."[2] I looked at the kettle and switched it on again. The button's orange light winked to show it was already working for me.

---

2. *Consciousness Can Be Quantified* by Michio Kaku, Big Think, 2014.

"Shall we do something about it?" I asked.

"Sure," said Gabriel, "what do you want to do?"

"Something. I want to do something." My creative thermostat switched on.

"You were just the same about other things you wanted to do," he said indifferently.

The kettle switched off, releasing thick steam that evaporated.

I took some mint from the fridge and washed it under a stream of water.

"But then I was only concerned with adding to our income; there was no choice. They weren't things I enjoyed doing. Now, I have something of my own to offer the world. And one day, when the boys are grown, I'll go back to painting," I said defensively.

I thrust clean mint leaves into a large glass without a handle.

"I don't even know how to convey this idea; it's so simple, so different. Best case scenario, people might think I'm crazy."

"If at first the idea is not absurd, then there is no hope for it"[3] responded Gabriel.

The slosh of boiling water being poured into the glass was soothing and filled my reflective mind. For myself, I prepared a white coffee: a mixture of coffee beans, ginger, cinnamon, cloves, and cardamom.

I returned to the living room with the hot drinks. "You know the people who say their work stems from a sense of calling and ideology; that they're less concerned with

---

3. A quote attributed to Einstein.

results? They claim that if only one person is touched, that's enough for them." I put his tea down on the table while holding onto my coffee. "That's how I feel. I simply have to do something about it; I feel as if I have no choice."

He nodded.

"Maybe I'll do a presentation on YouTube. It's a simple, easy tool for conveying information."

He blew on the tea and took a noisy sip. "Do a presentation." His response didn't satisfy me. I examined his face, wanting to get to the bottom of what he was thinking.

I sat down beside him. "You think I'm a lunatic, don't you? Otherwise, how come I know something no one else is aware of?"

"What do you think?"

"Listen, the whole idea is based on the heart's electromagnetic field. I didn't discover this. I only found another way to use it."

"Okay," he looked expectantly at me.

"Do you remember, years ago when we were still dating, there was a video on Facebook called "Healing the Heart?"[4] It was a rare documentary about a special hospital in China. It was a hospital that didn't use drugs. People were healed through energy. In the video, a woman lay on a bed and beside her was an ultrasound screen divided in two. On the left side – an image of a bladder with a malignant tumor seven centimeters in diameter, and on the right side – a live video of the tumor. Then, three practitioners who were trained to feel the process

---
4. From "Healing the Heart - an amazing lecture," 2007. Lecturer: Gregg Braden. YouTube Deep Truth Channel.

repeated the mantra: 'Was-sa,' 'Was-sa,' meaning "already happened". It sounded like a spiritual act of Voodoo taking place under the auspices of alternative medicine in order to make the malignancy vanish."

"I remember. I must admit it was incredible."

"As the practitioners whispered, you see the tumor beginning to contract, and after a few minutes, the malignant tumor became smaller and smaller until it had disappeared. The practitioners then applauded themselves."

"Yes, I remember."

"That video was only a small part of a three-hour lecture by Gregg Braden, the guy with the white hair, remember? Adele said he reminded her of Ori Hizkiah, a funny, interesting likeness between a stand-up comedian and a researcher of spiritual science."

Gabriel grinned.

"I listened to the lecture three times. I'd love to attend one of his lectures, even if it's overseas. Gregg Braden knows how to explain spiritual physics clearly, logically, and structurally; his words ignite the imagination and offer another aspect of natural world reality which suddenly appears fantastic, marvelous, and, primarily, very accessible."

"Is there any Bamba?"[5] asked Gabriel.

"And the video," I said loudly to keep him focused, "actually illustrates the human ability to use energy to make the tumor disappear; this is a documented medical procedure. All I'm talking about is the same kind of

---
5. A popular peanut butter puff snack in Israel.

aesthetic treatment that everybody has the power to do for themselves."

I waited several seconds for his response. I stared at him and he stared back.

"There are some small packets of Bamba," I said.

"So do a presentation, I dare you." Gabriel put his finger on the spinner and it revolved on its axis, enjoying the fulfillment of its calling.

Knowledge Sets Us Free

My own Butterfly Effect came from an unexpected source after reading a book that influenced me, gradually leading me to a shift in the worldview I'd consolidated over the years.

I was twenty-five when my whole world was turned upside down. I became the single parent of two beautiful, two-and-a-half-year-old infants. Unable to afford rent, I went back to live with my widowed father and had to look for a job that suited a young woman like myself, who had completed twelve years of schooling without full matriculation. Although I did have a medical secretary diploma, it was useless. The field meant shift work and I didn't have anyone to look after my little girls.

I was completely at a loss. One day, I was standing in the street talking to one of the mothers at the girls' daycare center and she recommended that I work as a cleaner. Smiling reassuringly at me, she waved her arms in all directions as if attempting to straighten out the air itself. She described the work as light and particularly glamorous, with short working hours and a high salary.

I had nothing to lose and decided to try. I found a small ad in the local newspaper and was quickly accepted for the job as a house cleaner, maybe because of my general, good-girl appearance. The owner of the house gave me a tour of the five-room duplex, which wasn't designed in a particularly original or exciting fashion, but, like the energy radiating from the tall, blond owner herself, it had a pleasant, warm, and quiet atmosphere. One of the rooms on the entrance floor served as a small office. In it was a table, a computer, and a modest library on two shelves. I scanned it with great interest. She apparently noticed my curiosity and generously offered to lend me books.

I worked mornings three times a week. I had my own key and when I entered the apartment, I'd say "hello" to the large, colorful parrot thoughtlessly spitting seed shells out of its cage. I turned the television onto the Israeli music channel. I washed the dishes by hand even though there was a dishwasher in the kitchen, removed mugs with coffee dregs from the bathroom, and carried out all sorts of routine tasks.

One morning, while dusting the little office with pink cloth, the books caught my attention and called me to examine them. Most of the books were about marketing, but there were a few novels. I only found one book that looked rather interesting to me and I liked its name: *Universe on a T-Shirt*.[6] I pulled it out. It was a book about the history of physics from Ancient Greece to the present day. I knew nothing about physics; we didn't study physics in high school, and I didn't know anything about it. My general notion of physics was that it was a sophisticated subject intended for seriously brainy people with degrees who love numbers, formulas and equations. I knew that

---

6. By Dan Falk, translated by: Shlomit Kna'an, Keter Publishing House, 2005.

physics was connected to the *theory of relativity* and a genius with wild, white hair who stuck out his tongue. The book was new and it was published that year. On the back cover I read that it got its name after scientists were challenged to find one elegant formula that would unify all universal forces in one simple equation. It was written that the book was meant for everyone, even those with no understanding of physics. I thought that the book was perfect for me, and I decided to borrow it.

I didn't know at the time that I would also find a common denominator and unifier among things that appear unrelated to each other. This ultimately, would make me challenge conventional thinking on the subject of permanent hair removal.

"The God Particle"

It was Saturday night. My little girls were asleep in their beds in a small housing unit in my father's large villa. It was dark and quiet outside and a faint light shone from the kitchen. Sitting on the edge of my bed, I leaned my elbows on my knees and summed up my impression of the fascinating book that had exposed me to all kinds of people I'd never before encountered. They were people who devoted and are still devoting their time to searching for the largest variety of physical phenomena in the world in order to find a common denominator. They took an interest in the nature of the universe. They observed the earth, plants, stars, and life's great abundance, wondering how and from what material the world was created. I had never thought so deeply. I'd never considered the question of the source of things around me. If it weren't for the interesting stories in the book and figures I'd previously encountered only by name, like Tycho Brahe, Galileo, and Newton, I might easily have thought they were people who had no life of their own.

In time, prompted by the curiosity of such people, great progress was made by mentally peeling away layers of matter. As a result of modern technological development, science can now see active atomic space. People with brilliant minds have managed to simplify the understanding of matter so that today we don't need to know advanced placement-level physics in order to have a general idea of how the world works. Anyone can understand and enjoy the disseminated wisdom of geniuses and the workings of the Divine in matter.

One chapter of the book echoed in my mind: a concise explanation of "string theory." Inherent in the theory is the hope of unifying all the mysterious forces active in the universe which, apparently, consists of a unified field of strings. The strings are active deep within the atom, vibrating and creating frequency waves like the strings of a violin. The universe is a live music concert, played by sounds from infinite strings becoming different textures of matter. The size of a string in relation to the body is the size of a tree in relation to the universe.

I was raised to believe that God is everywhere and that nothing can exist in reality without His presence; there is none other but Him. It has been scientifically proven that the "divine code" is in our DNA.

"God dwells in us, and we in Him."

I closed my eyes in order to reach the edge of the universe within me - the strings. In my mind, I launched myself straight to the front of a single, impressive cell. I penetrated the thin crust surrounding it, finding myself in a round warm pool of organelles like jelly candies. Tiny, round, white spheres of matter circled around me, as if I were inside a magnificent, live snowball. I dove into the depths of the great cell nucleus. A pair of misty blue-purple chromosomes moved slowly. Inside them, I was dwarfed by a coiled double helix of DNA - and then, darkness spread swiftly and completely.

In the distance, a tiny atom glitters like a star and, close by, electrons revolve around the atom in non-stop elliptical circles, leaving behind a cloudy trail. I penetrated the atom and the neutron particle. Minuscule quark particles floated in the depths of space like fireflies and, passing into the quark, I felt myself moving at an ever-increasing pace. Without points of reference, I flew through the dark for a time until I no longer knew where or if I was moving at all. I couldn't orient myself in space without a sense of self, time was like a clock that had lost its hands. I didn't know how to continue to navigate my being; I was lost in internal space. I considered giving up the quest. But then, a distant flash of sparks instilled its presence in me. I had reached my destination. I was face to face with strings in a myriad of colors like slender, unsymmetrical hoops of light moving in a joyful, dance-like rhythm. I was mesmerized by their movement until I felt comfortable enough to open my eyes in my familiar room.

I was awed by the concept of God dwelling deep inside my body, strumming my strings and making sure they were always tuned to the right frequency. I sensed the "touch" of God and knew I wasn't ever alone. He was part of me, always with me – every moment of my life.

He was the quiet presence of a hidden, protective, and loving strength inside me.

I was moved and stunned by the closeness of the Divine and large, warm and utterly unexpected tears flowed down my cheeks. The front door opened. My sister-in-law, dressed in black, stood on the threshold. She looked at me with concern, frowned, and asked, "what's wrong?" I didn't know how to explain what I was feeling, and I wasn't sure if it would interest her, so I responded: "I'm not sad." I wiped away the tears and went towards her.

The philosopher Albert Camus said: "Live to the point of tears." This was my point of tears. Here, I found whom my soul loves: the world of theoretical physics.

I searched for more information in the large library I used to visit as a little girl in elementary school. A large sign hung high between the bookshelves:

"If You Read, It Will Happen."

I was impressed by the sentence, though I didn't entirely understand what it meant and wondered to myself what could happen.

I borrowed books on physics from Einstein's time, books on special relativity and quantum physics theory. I very quickly found myself drawn to this unique field. The field explains the atom as a particle of matter that also behaves like a wave of energy.

I came up with my understanding:

Quantum particles defy convention and violate the law of Newton in whose world there is no room for change and life travels a repetitive path similar to our daily routine. But, at the heart of matter are tiny, mysterious, swift, elusive, and weird quantum particles. They are characterized by uncertainty, spontaneous adventure, energy, and joy of life, and they can be defined as "little guys" that like to test the boundaries of their ability to experience, simultaneously, all possibilities in reality.

If, for instance, a quantum particle was the size of a person, you could arrange to meet him. However, you would have to take into account that he would have other meetings at all possible times, present, past and future, and there would only be a probable chance of his arrival. When he sets out, he penetrates the doors of his hybrid vehicle and travels the freeway in all directions at once. If we know his location on the way, we cannot predict his speed, and if we know how fast he travels, we cannot know for certain where he is.

The human particle behaves like a complex double agent that is able to be in several places at once. In the sea, for instance, surfing the waves of opportunity. If we find and observe him, even from a distance, we are also able to see him on the beach, walking along the sand like an ordinary person. Scientists were puzzled by what appeared to be a totally chaotic set of particles that do not provide simple, logical answers for their behavior. Scientists tried hard to find order in the chaos and lost themselves in the process.

"If you aren't confused by quantum mechanics, you haven't really understood it," said Professor Nils Bohr, while his friend, Professor Einstein, also a pioneer in quantum theory, found it hard to believe in the unstable nature of particles. In a letter to Nils Bohr, he wrote that "God does not play dice with the universe." His friend responded "don't tell God what to do." Out of all this, the only thing I was certain about was that these little guys seriously affected me and that their world is my world. They are part of my body and so I should know more about them in order to connect with their unique powers. Maybe then, I'd be able to influence my life, change conventions in my ordinary world and be a kind of Wonder Woman in the world of particles within me.

Theory

Seven years went by during which I read books and watched documentary films on theoretical physics. Physics thrilled me, filling me with a passion to know more.

I was busy trying to tidy the little house on a boiling summer day, about two hours before the girls were due home from school. On the computer was the documentary film, *What the Bleep Do We Know*, which deals with quantum theory. I'd seen the film before so I just listened to it. It was like background music of enthusiastic physics professors. And like any description of unexpected enlightenment that occurs in the flash of one moment in time, this is also what happened to me when I heard the sentence:

"Each cell in the body has a consciousness."[7]

The sentence was powerfully heard in my mind, causing an overflow of information about plants, which are also said to have consciousness. I remembered experiments carried out on plants during which they were spoken to with negative energy, which caused them to dry

---

[7]. From the documentary "What the Bleep Do We Know" (2004).

up and wither. And then a picture formed in my mind: dry body hair like withered leaves.

This made me think it possible to affect body hair, causing it to dry up, wither, and stop growing. This is due to the significant internal common denominator of plants and body cells: consciousness. Or, in the ancient words: "for man is like the tree of the field."[8]

First, the connection between things amuses me. However, it was clear to me that this was a real and serious idea that could manifest. The impossible is relative to what the mind has prepared itself to understand, grasp, and see, but everything is subject to the laws of nature, which are actually rather flexible.

I thought about the film "The Secret" and how quite a few people already know the power of thought and that it is possible to influence the body. There are people who know it is possible to remove hair energetically through talking or some similar act. It isn't that anyone is waiting for me to say something, and maybe I'm the last one to know about it. In addition, I had no interest in trying, primarily because at the time, permanent hair removal wasn't a crucial need for me. Other things preoccupied me: I was at the beginning of a relationship with a man fourteen years older than me. In time, he became my husband.

About eight months after we met, Gabriel and I had a small and modest ceremony in an apartment he'd rented. We had two witnesses and a ring, in accordance with the Law of Moses and Israel.

---

8. Deuteronomy 20:19.

The following day, the girls and I went to live in his home on a small Moshav[9] in central Israel.

Once we'd settled in on the Moshav, I remembered my theory about hair and stopping its growth, and I felt the desire to try and examine it in reality. However, my spirit animal is a sloth and, as usual, I procrastinated. Then, I discovered I was pregnant and knew I shouldn't talk to my body with the intention of influencing it during pregnancy, because the fetus is conscious of its mother's feelings and shouldn't be part of a journey of questions and talking about permanent hair removal, even if it's a sweet little female fetus with particularly hairy genes. Apart from that, during pregnancy a woman's hair grows at a more moderate pace because her body focuses most of its energy on the developing fetus and less on trivialities like hair growth.

After my sweet boy was born, I wasn't free to contend with my theory. Naturally, all my energy was focused on him, to say nothing of the fact that I was a gifted procrastinator. So, I invented a distant, unpredictable goal: the end of my next pregnancy. In the meantime, life on the little Moshav was rather limited, even for someone like me who doesn't usually spend much time outside. I desperately needed to move to the city and, two weeks before my second birth, when Ethan was one and a half years old, we moved away to an apartment about a twenty minutes' drive north of a city with the biggest power plant. It is a "city of energy" – a living place.

---

9. A moshav is a type of Israeli town or settlement; a type of cooperative agricultural community of individual farms.

We moved to an old, three-room apartment intended for an evacuation-construction project, located parallel to the main street in the Ha-Otsar neighborhood. 'Otsar' means 'treasure.' Although the apartment was small, we chose it because we liked its interior; it was full of light.

The Presentation

After updating Gabriel on my personal development and the little hair experiment I conducted, I was certain I was in possession of important information, especially after hearing nothing about this concept for years. I imagined there'd probably be a handful of people who'd be glad to know about it and who would appreciate the information. I was determined to spread the idea. I felt an inexplicable urge as if the destiny of ethical hair treatment lay in my hands. So, in the evenings after my small boys had fallen asleep, I sat on my computer in front of the PowerPoint program.

"What are you doing?" Adele, my fourteen-year-old daughter, stood beside me, gazing at the screen with interest.

"Drafting a presentation on talking to hair. But I'm no expert on presentations."

"What will you do with it?"

"Upload it to YouTube." Oh Lord, help!

"Like I wanted to open a channel?"

"No, my lovely. You wanted to open a makeup channel to demonstrate how you make up your eyes and powder your button of a nose, just like a lot of young girls who don't understand very much about makeup. You weren't old enough to do it and certainly couldn't lecture or explain it like a professional makeup artist."

"I was thirteen," she protested.

"Exactly. Could you make me a coffee, please," I said, terminating the conversation.

The entrance door rubbed against the floor and a slight scrape was heard, signaling the best part of the day: Gabriel had arrived and I could talk to a handsome adult again.

Gabriel entered the house with Donald Trump, the new President of the United States. The President's loud voice was coming out of the smartphone he held in his hand.

"Want to see?" I instantly called out.

He stopped the President's speech, put his black leather bag on the small table in the kitchen, and came towards me.

"See what?"

"I've finished the presentation. I've written the theory and I must have made too many transitions and animations because it looks like a word cartoon."

I enlarged the screen and for about a minute we gazed at revolving windows and jumping white print on a black background.

"I have a theory based on facts and a hypothesis, but nobody will take what I've written seriously." I was frustrated. "I have great information and no idea of how to get it across. It's professionally feeble. The presentation is childish and mostly insipid. I can't possibly upload it to YouTube in its present form."

I apologized, primarily to myself.

"Keep working on it," said Gabriel, and he went to see if he could rustle up something to eat in the kitchen.

I raised my voice: "But I don't know anything about presentations or YouTube, and I don't feel like knowing anything about it. I'm not a technological type, even if it's supposed to be simple. It's complicated for me."

Gabriel was already in the kitchen, more attentive to the sounds of his belly than to me.

"Your coffee's ready," said Adele on her way to her room. "Thank you," I said, hoping she'd put in too much sugar. I got up and turned to Gabriel, comforted by the fact that I was doing all that I could.

I continued to work on the presentation in the evenings, pretending it was going somewhere.

The Guide

When Gabriel came in that morning, he'd obviously had a haircut. His short beard was trimmed close to his cheeks. The rimless glasses on his eyes seemed cleaner; or was this an optical illusion due to the neat style of his beard?

"Someone I met at the barber is on his way here. I told him you have an interesting theory. He distributes products on the Internet, and he can help you."

"How symbolic: to find someone who can help promote the concept of hair removal in a barber shop," I said, feeling skeptical.

Gabriel had already disappeared down the passage.

Tom, my little one-and-a-half-year-old son, was pushing a tiny blue car along the floor tiles in the living room. He came over to me, saying slowly, "Mummy, h-a-air!" He held out two fingers to which clung a single strand of long dark hair. He didn't know what to do with it and I was aware that from a young age, he perceived hair as something disgusting. It took me a few seconds to get a hold of the fine hair and I shook it off my fingers. I let it drop to the floor; it was unnecessary to accompany it on its final journey to the garbage. Tom calmed down and tugged at his ear. He returned to his game, making the sounds of a little car now rolling along the table. Nearby, Ethan played with a green car.

"He's on his way," said Gabriel, who appeared in the living room and hinted at the mess.

I tidied up the games that were spread over the floor, although I realized rather quickly that I was only moving some of the toys from one side of the room to the other.

There was a knock at the door. Gabriel went to open it and on the threshold stood a young man who seemed hesitant or reluctant at the spontaneous encounter in a stranger's home.

"I'm glad you came," Gabriel welcomed him.

The man entered and saw me.

"Hello," I smiled at him, gesturing to him to sit on the sofa.

"Hello," he responded formally, and took two long steps before sitting down alertly on the sofa.

"What's your name?" I asked.

"Arik, pleased to meet you."

"Pleased to meet you," I responded, continuing to stand.

"Your husband told me you have an idea you want to market on the internet."

I hadn't thought about marketing, but it sounded good. "What is it that you do exactly?"

"I have a website where I sell products." He seemed to be feeling more comfortable.

"Like what?"

"All sorts of things, like stickers for radiation protection from smartphones and a patent for German fuel-saving technology."

"Sounds interesting," I nodded. What could I possibly

say about products I'd never heard of? "I tried marketing on eBay, but it's not for me."

"It's different because I have my own website. Tell me about your idea."

"I've discovered a way to remove hair permanently."

"How does it work?"

I briefly explained the facts and my theory. His face remained expressionless. I tried to work out what he was thinking, and he didn't ask if it worked. He might have respected the personal issue with its aspect of privacy.

"You could write a twenty-page guide and I'll market it cheaply on the internet."

I was amazed; I hadn't thought of it like that and it was so obvious: just write a guide.

"Digital guides are a basic product and are quite normal overseas," added Arik, when I didn't react.

"I didn't know," I responded, feeling like a first-grade student who had received homework for the first time.

"I'm in touch with the coach, Alon Gal. I listen to his radio program every Friday. People call in and get advice from him. Wait, I'll play it for you. Last Friday, he spoke to a woman who invented a method of treating teeth after she'd suffered a great deal. She accumulated a great amount of knowledge over the years, collecting and correlating data until she arrived at a formula she successfully tried on herself and wanted to make public."

"Rather like myself."

He fiddled with his smartphone and began to play me the recording of Alon Gal's broadcast, but I didn't get the point even after listening attentively for several minutes.

"To make it short, he told her to prepare a guide and sell it," Arik summarized.

I gained the impression he was a sincere, honest person. I thought he possessed the energy to climb the ladder of success.

"I also advertise products on Facebook. Do you want to see it?"

I didn't. I understood what I had to do and the meeting was at an end as far as I was concerned. I saw no point in examining various products and, in any case, Gabriel and I aren't a target audience for purchasing unnecessary gadgets.

"So I'll write something and get back to you?"

"Yes, great. Approximately two months?"

"Yes," I replied.

"Good, so we'll be in touch," Arik concluded. He looked at Gabriel and got to his feet.

"Thank you," I said.

When the door closed behind him, I immediately thought of the next step.

"I'm not sure whether I have enough information on the subject. I only have the gist of a theory and barely any experience. But I could try; I do have general knowledge regarding theoretical physics."

"Go ahead, write a guide," said Gabriel encouragingly.

Ethan approached his father and gestured to him to pick him up. Gabriel lifted him. Ethan, who noticed the change in his father's face, stroked his trimmed beard.

"Thorns!" Alarmed, he leaned back, wrinkling his nose and rubbing his hands.

"Bristles," Gabriel laughingly corrected him, and tossed him into the air.

A Pink Mustache

"Do you really think I could be happy?!" A curious Bergen with a yellow mustache asked Poppy, the pink troll.

"Of course, it's inside you! It's inside all of us, and I don't think it, I feel it!" Cried Poppy excitedly, smiling at the Bergens who were standing around the table on which she stood. The opening music of the song "Can't Stop the Feeling"[10] played and Poppy began to sing and dance.

The clip played in the background. The song filled me with an inspired rhythm. As I typed my words, I discovered an enjoyment rather than the boredom of producing a presentation. However, when the song ended, I found myself drumming my fingers on the table, stuck in front of the screen without words.

I lacked experience. I decided to start the process from the beginning and take care of my mustache hair. This is facial hair that most women remove, and so I thought it appropriate to write about the process of energetically removing mustache hair.

I took a sheet of paper from the printer next to the computer and after several attempts to write the heading

---

10. "Can't Stop the Feeling." Official Movie Clip – Trolls 5. DreamWorksTV by Peacock Kids.

"MUSTACHE" at the top of the page with cheap blue pens that didn't work, I noticed a pink marker just waiting to be chosen. My artistic side offered an alternative: instead of writing, I took the marker and, at the top of the page, I drew a thick pink masculine mustache with curled ends. I cello-taped the page next to the mirror in the bathroom so that I could mark each time I did a treatment and could keep track of the number of treatments. I made sure to close the door so that I had complete privacy. I was aware that my older girls could hear me talking to the mustache, because their room was in the middle of the short passage near the bathroom. I tried not to let this distract me. However, this was no ordinary activity for me either, and I knew I was crossing the boundaries of what was considered sane and normal. I assumed that this was what people would think when people talk to plants.

I had no doubt that this was the right and best way to connect my external world with the inner, hypothetical world in order to influence it. I focused on the thought that in my opinion it was a logical act and it didn't matter if it was uncommon for others.

The plucking ritual included a spool of black sewing thread and I had to rip off a piece of it each time. I made sure that the thread was neither too long nor too short so that I could hold it comfortably and make a tiny knot that connected the two edges.

I looked in the mirror framed with a yellowish plastic strip connected to a matching, narrow, plastic shelf.

I didn't like my hair and I didn't know how or if it was possible to enjoy the process.

I took a deep breath and began to command my hair, "stop growing."

I examined it close up. It didn't seem to make an impression.

"Stop growing." A stuttering sound came from my throat.

Embarrassed, I cleared it.

I thought I should start talking, if only technically at first, just to convey the information that the hair had to stop growing.

I uttered the sentence like a mantra, so that the feeling would accompany it naturally, or so I believed.

"Stop growing." I directly addressed the hair on the left and plucked it out with the thread.

"Stop growing." I said, and felt myself getting angry. I plucked the stray hairs.

I imagined the hairs had ears.

"Stop growing." I ordered, not really sure it wanted to listen to me.

"Stop growing." It has to do as I say. I plucked.

"Stop growing." I'll force it.

"Stop growing." I'm the one who decides. I plucked its presence.

"Stop growing." Irritating hair. I plucked its impertinence.

"Stop growing." I glared at it.

"Stop growing." I didn't know what it thought of me.

"Stop growing." I didn't know what I was meant to feel.

"Stop growing." If only I had a guide.

I felt frustrated, strange, and weak opposite the protein threads doing whatever they wanted inside me.

Nonetheless, I repeated the mantra again and again until I finished the treatment and my upper lip was hairless.

I blinked at my reflection in the mirror. I wasn't pleased with my emotional process during the hair treatment. I felt that happiness came with anger and that I needed to exercise an unnatural authority that didn't even fully convince me. It wasn't easy for me to convey the message to the hair. The stress and lack of confidence in my strength and authority confused me, and the general sensation was unpleasant, to say the least.

I'd never had a managerial position, so the experience of giving an order wasn't exactly one of my strengths. Maybe that was an excuse. But one thing was clear to me: since it was my hair, I had to make the decision. I was its guardian even without a legal court document. All the authority in the process was in my power.

Hopefully, I'd know how to upgrade and perfect the process in time.

The part I did enjoy came at the end of the treatment, when I wrote the date on the page under the drawing of the mustache.

I wondered how come I hadn't talked to my mustache before when it was ostensibly the first area to treat. After all, facial hair was exposed and required regular removal. How come I hadn't thought of doing it right from the beginning, when I first started energetically treating my hair?

I tried to think of whom to discuss it with, and I knew I had no partner in this subject.

The mirror on the wall looked at me. If I talked to the mirror, would it answer me? I wouldn't ask it who is the fairest of them all[11]; that didn't particularly interest me.

My question would be: Mirror, mirror on the wall, who is the sanest of them all on the issue of hair removal methods?

---

11. The tale of "Snow White and the Seven Dwarfs" by the Grimm Brothers.

External Research

I began to watch YouTube videos about hair removal, curious about the different takes on the subject. I was surprised to see a large number of videos. Every day another video on the subject was uploaded.

This included vlogs by women who do laser hair removal treatments and women who oppose laser treatments, the challenges of waxing for men, video on a hundred years of hair removal techniques, young girls who demonstrate how to shave facial hair, experiences and opinions regarding new technological products for hair removal, and a woman who explores twenty-one hair removal methods on both her legs.

I was exposed to a reality where the main feeling was that of pain and frustration. I was unaware of the magnitude of the predicament, and could not have imagined just how difficult life with ostensibly unnecessary hair could be for both men and women.

I was absorbed in what had appeared on the computer screen when Adele addressed me: "aren't you tired of watching videos on hair removal?"

"It's interesting. I've realized that hair removal is considered a nightmare for everyone. Period. Everyone goes through the torture chamber of hair removal and, even if the majority only shave, this has side effects of itching, sores, and hair growth under the skin."

"Ugh, Mom," Adele said, revolted, "that's disgusting."

"I watched Indian girls. They are undoubtedly the princesses of hair removal videos. Many Indian women suffer from excessive hair. They use natural ingredients found in any kitchen to prepare various hair removal concoctions which are endlessly demonstrated in the videos."

"That stuff doesn't work," stated Adele with complete certainty.

"I've just seen a video about someone who recommended leaving the natural concoction on the body all night."

"For hair made of steel wool?" asked Adele cynically.

I quickly typed into the search bar: **"Hair removal forum."** Most people try to get some idea about the problem through searching for symptoms on the internet. Doctor Google refers people to forums joined by professional doctors or ordinary people with personal experience. "Listen," I read from the computer: **"Is it advisable to remove hair from the arms by shaving? Won't the hair grow back darker?"**

"Do we need epilation to remove hair from sideburns and the chin? Isn't there something less painful and safer? I've heard it can leave scars." Adele's face was a mixture of wonder and pity.

"That's nothing; remember Harnaam Kaur?"

"No," she answered after trying to remember.

"Guinness World Records, 2017, the youngest bearded woman."

"Yes, oy, shocking."

"She doesn't find it shocking to have a full beard. I think she's beautiful with her beard and perfect, full, red lips. Her beard seems to suit her and, maybe, if she didn't have a beard, she'd feel something was missing from her face. Maybe she'd have stuck a false beard onto herself."

"That would drive me nuts."

"There are quite a few women with full beards who feel beautiful and unique. Maybe this is because a beard isn't only a phenomenon among hairy women. The full beard gives a different kind of character to women who, at a certain stage of maturity and after years of frustration with the never-ending struggle to remove it, adopt their unique appearance with love."

"Whatever," said Adele dismissively.

"You're still growing up. But it's important to know that in young girls, excessive hairiness stems from a hormonal imbalance known as Polycystic Ovarian Syndrome.'"

Adele stared at the screen. She didn't want to hear about illness. There was no point in trying to interest her in extreme situations of hair growth. I continued to read about the common problems of hair removal:

"If I remove hair from my nose, won't the hair grow back longer?"

"I have a lot of hair on my forehead; how can I get rid of it?"

"Help me – I'm going nuts. Unfortunately, I am very hairy. I'm willing to endure a lot of pain, but my

hair grows back too quickly. I don't know what to do with my hair anymore. Never mind my arms, legs, and belly, what about the bush and butt hair? What the hell do I do about that?!"

Adele's jaw dropped. "TMI" she instinctively blurted out.

"When I first started writing about energetic hair removal, I really didn't think it through," I sighed. "Of course, I can't write an entire guide about hair removal without mentioning these important places and giving them their due," I said.

"Mom, that is so embarrassing," said Adele, revolted.

"Yes, but those are intimate places. The question of whether or not to remove hair there is controversial. I don't have to take a stand on the issue; I only bring factual data and offer help, which is a perfectly natural solution for anyone who is interested or deliberating."

"I don't envy you." Adele shook her head and walked off.

I was left with my thoughts.

Private areas of the body occasionally require medical examination, whereupon it is relatively easy to overcome the embarrassment caused by a qualified practitioner's examination when it relates to health. However, in my opinion, if hair is the problem, this is merely an aesthetic issue and the embarrassment is greater. Even if the practitioner qualified to remove hair is exposed daily to the sight of intimate organs, this is no comfort to the patient and it does not alleviate the sense of personal exposure. The fact that it doesn't occur to women and men that they can permanently and privately rid themselves of hair in these areas arouses distress and helplessness. It bothered me that people behave as if they need nursing care in an aesthetic field.

After watching a considerable number of videos, the value of energetic hair removal became clearer to me and it strengthened my desire to take part in providing a suitable solution to the problem.

I came to the conclusion that most products, techniques, and patents that exist on the market don't really offer a satisfactory or perfect answer for long-lasting hair-free skin.

We gift the industry the power and responsibility of nurturing us when we rely too much on products and technology that cannot do the wonderful, beautiful work that the body can do on its own in private, without the need for an appointment with a practitioner and without side effects in a manner that is perfectly adapted to individual body hair.

Hair doesn't grow with the help of special devices external to the body. Therefore, in order to stop the act of growth, it makes sense to reverse the same natural growth mechanism to implement a fundamental core treatment. This would occur without the devices and aids we are familiar with: tweezers, razors, wax, creams, electric shavers, epilation, laser, light, and even sound waves. Entire shelves, departments, and large stores are devoted to the subject. Further enhancements of devices and patents are constantly developed and offered to the public under the banner of good news and the notion that these will help us remove hair with maximum ease and comfort.

The widespread use of electrical equipment for the treatment of delicate cells in the body such as hair follicles is perceived as technological progress, but actually it is primitive in terms of the significance of hair and our personal relationship with it.

True, most equipment does the job. The real problem is not in the products themselves but in the dependence they foster, which is a dependence that continues throughout one's life and induces people to look outside for help. No one has ever taught us the power of favorably helping ourselves to change a situation. We should not only react to growing hair but actively treat it by ourselves. The wonderful experience of treating oneself facilitates flexibility and a shift in perspective.

It isn't fair that we are born with soft downy hair all over our body which, with the cruelty of puberty, grows and darkens, putting down strong roots and declaring its seemingly stubborn presence as if, time after time, it were clinging to our body and refusing to surrender. It is hair that leads us into a very long and tiring struggle accompanied by the eternal question of who will win. Even the brief peace that exists in us while our skin is hairless is always accompanied by dissatisfaction, because we know that the hair is already taking its first determined steps towards regrowth.

An Experiment that Went Wrong

The follow-up chart in the bathroom indicated that ten weeks and ten treatments had passed during which I'd held intense, expectant talks with my mustache. However, a close inspection in the mirror of the length, thickness, and lightness of the hair showed that no change had taken place. No reaction. No response. The commands had not been carried out, and the mustache was still dark and dense. I was disappointed. Why wasn't it working? Why wasn't the hair responding? Was my mustache deaf? Was it an anarchist? Could it be different from the other areas of my body? Was my theory completely incorrect? Was it incomplete? Should I wait until I succeed with the experiment to write the guide or should I simply give up?

    I tried to understand what had gone wrong. After devoting several days to concentrated thought, I decided to relax and allow the answer to come to me. Inviting it in, I trusted that the thought would come. Since the issue was important to me, I felt it would be a pity to waste time on despair, and I was willing to wait patiently for the right moment to bring an answer.

As far as I was concerned, it was okay not to know everything at once. I believed that delay was a necessary part of the developing experiment process. The stage of impasse and uncertainty is surely experienced by every researcher.

A Little Girl

Gabriel called to me from the kitchen: "Arik sent me a text message asking what's happening and whether you've finished writing the guide."

"I'm not sure about working with him," I responded. I was at the computer.

"Why not?"

"Because it doesn't feel right to me. Tell him it will take me a long time to write it," it was an excuse, but I had no other response and, in any case, it seemed as though I hadn't thought it through. To write a guide for such a different concept about a process in an unknown experiment isn't something one does within two months.

I wanted to share with Gabriel the universal difficulty of removing hair.

"Hey, I'm reading about the history of hair removal online, are you listening?"

Gabriel didn't respond, so I assumed he was.

"Ever since ancient Egypt, men and women have struggled with the removal of body hair. They used shells, tweezers, and a stone sponge to rub the hair. They also used sugar to form a type of wax just as they do today. Even then they used that technique. In the days of the

Roman Empire, they used flint and creams to remove unwanted hair. The wealthy classes could be identified by their hairless bodies. Statues of the Gods and paintings of women from the upper classes were all hairless."

"In that case, everyone in this generation belongs to the upper class," commented Gabriel, at once raising the status of humanity.

"Quality of life undoubtedly increases with the advance of technology. Notice that the first shaving device and hair removal cream for women was invented in 1915. During the forties', after the Second World War, there was a shortage of nylon stockings and women were forced to go bare-legged. They had to take care of their legs and an electric shaver was invented."

I got up and went to Gabriel.

"From everything I've read, it seems that a method has been repeated throughout human history; it is the method of rubbing hair with stones, resulting in 'shell shocked' skin. Imagine how much strength it would take to endure pain like that." I sat down opposite Gabriel who was eating onion soup with parmesan.

"There's a sentence: *Il faut souffrir pour être belle*."

"What does it mean?"

He looked gravely at me and responded, "one has to suffer to be beautiful."

I was exhilarated.

"That's exactly what my elder sister told me the first time she removed my mustache, and it hurt so much I'd barely let her do it. She made me believe that one has to suffer.

How can a twelve-year-old girl argue with a long

tradition of women suffering in the belief that this is the only way? It must be a universal expression that could certainly be considered as passing the torch of pain from mother to daughter in order to maintain restraint and self-respect through physical sacrifice and a passion for external beauty. Maybe it's all about the desire to feel good about ourselves and the need to show off to others in order to get their approval of our existence."

"But you're not like that, are you?"

I hesitated briefly. "I'm not sure about that. The need to look beautiful is in my female genes. The fact is that after my sister removed my mustache, the first thing I did was to go to my neighbor Yael to show her that I looked better. I wanted to brag and I beamed when she complimented me. Even today, after I remove the mustache…"

I fell silent.

Flashes illuminated my brain and a network of neurons connected my past experience with the present.

I had my answer. It came to me. I realized why I hadn't succeeded with my mustache; it was so clear and simple. I was filled with a peaceful energy.

Gabriel stared at me.

"I finally get it," I said, as a large smile spread across my face.

"You do? What?"

I linked my fingers and wondered how to explain it without being awkward.

"I had a problem removing the hair on my upper lip and now I realize why. When I talked to my mustache, I didn't really intend for it to stop growing because the memory of feeling so special after my neighbor's compliment is preserved in my subconscious. My inner child resisted. She didn't want me to have a smooth upper lip forever because then she wouldn't experience that wonderful clean sensation whenever I, the adult, remove the mustache. I now realize that I was addicted to that feeling and didn't know it."

"The treatment failed? It didn't work?" Gabriel didn't sound surprised.

"My treatment is fine," I hurried to clarify, "the problem lay in my subconscious, emotional response, which I'm supposed to change."

Gabriel lost interest. Getting up, he cleared the table and went into the living room. I followed him, forcing him to listen to me as if he were my bestie.

He picked up heavy metal Chinese balls that lay in a round, woven basket on the table among tiny cars and a small blunt pencil. Lolling on the sofa, he expertly rolled the balls in his large, masculine hand. I stood in front of him.

"I read on the internet[12] about Rebecca Herzig, an American writer and researcher who wrote the book: 'Plucked: A History of Hair Removal'. The article about the book reveals some of the extreme hair removal methods from the past. You wouldn't believe the mad age-old conflict between people and their body hair. It is a struggle that developed into a massacre with every possible means used to get rid of hair. The most shocking thing was that during the sixties', women used a cream containing rat poison to remove hair.

---

12. Based on: Meitar Schleider Putschnik, "Dying Smoothly: The Deadly History of Hair Removal," 15.2.2017, News!

This caused muscular dystrophy, blindness, and death. It's horrifying to discover the lengths to which women were willing to go out of despair and an obsession with beauty. It all came from a lack of knowledge about the properties of the substance and the nature of hair."

"You're overdoing it," declared Gabriel, ostentatiously turning the balls in his hand. I sat down next to him. "I'm explaining it to you. At the time, doctors treated Hirsutism – that was the medical term for excess hair growth – as if it were a disease. It gave doctors an excuse to prescribe hormonal medication that is today used to treat transgender individuals. The side effects caused cancer, strokes, and heart attacks."

"Horrifying."

"Yes. Throughout history, people have tried to find solutions with the same superficial thinking that hair should be removed by forceful, violent, and external means in order for it to be destroyed. It's sad that the general human perception is that in life we have to fight for everything we want to achieve, when in truth all wars are ultimately won within ourselves. If war is the approach, then the best strategy is to subdue the enemy without a struggle. When removing hair energetically it's easy to understand the 'enemy,' the simple perspective of hair, which can make it stop growing on its own without the tools of war on a battlefield."

Gabriel listened attentively.

"The answer is much simpler. It is available and today we have the appropriate knowledge and spiritual preparation. Our generation is ready for spiritual ideas as effective treatments for the body. As I see it, it seems mad to relate only to the external, physical layer of the body."

Gabriel's eyes narrowed in suspicion. "Haven't you ever done anything crazy for beauty's sake? You are, after all, a woman." He continued to turn the balls swiftly to improve the flexibility of his fingers.

I had to prove to myself that I wasn't crazy. Leaning back, I went through my memory library, trying to find a sane documented act that I didn't believe would yield fruit. Then, I found it. A single memory, from the age of twenty-one, was thrust among tiny cells. I was obsessed with trying to remove a specific mole from the middle of my left arm from which one, long, dark hair protruded.

The obsession, inaction, and temporary disconnection from all common sense came together to make me believe that this was the most crucial thing in the world and that I had to take care of it without delay. I took an extremely strong cleaning liquid intended for cleaning toilets and spread it on the mole with the help of a Q-tip. It burned fiercely but I didn't care. It was important to me that the mole disappear and that the long hair would stop growing. The area quickly became red and itchy and I felt the substance "eating" my skin. At that point, I woke up and realized that this was stupid and abnormal. I ran to wash my arm under the tap. A burn resulted and actually it wasn't worth it; the mole became clearer and the hair grows to this day. As a souvenir, I have a small scar.

I did it to myself. I deliberately hurt my body. As far as I'm concerned it was a sin. I looked at the scar and covered it with my palm. Does every woman experience a moment like this?

There was no point in trying to explain something that wasn't entirely clear to me and never happened again.

"Something crazy?" I responded, protecting my past. "I would never invest in the external at the expense of the spiritual." It was true.

Gabriel nodded.

"I have always preferred to buy a book than new pants," I added.

"Actually, it would be nice if you'd buy a pretty skirt; you don't know how to dress."

"Buying a book is a lot easier."

"Undoubtedly. You're not a woman in every sense of the word."

I resented his comment. "I am. I'm just not constantly preoccupied with my appearance."

Routine

As a homemaker and full-time mom, I took care of my kids, made food, shopped, ran errands, and took them to the playground, park, and the library.

I played, laughed, got mad and tired, made more food, bathed them, and read a bedtime story. Sometimes I even read two or three.

I sat in front of the computer and drank a cup of coffee or two or three. I found words inside me, typed, and formed sentences. The sound of typing reminded me of a word factory, one that sketches a map of insight for a hidden but easily accessible world. There was a new and wonderful experience I'd hoped people would want to discover to try and surprise themselves in an adventure with a hairless body and a beauty already intrinsic to them.

Every day, I ate, drank, and breathed stopping the growth of hair through energy talking. I persistently wrote about it and at night as I fell asleep I continued to think about it.

I wondered how one should really talk to hair. How does one convey such a different idea to different people? What situations were people likely to encounter? Would some people prefer to practice through meditation?

What was the right frequency for such treatments? What constitutes hair consciousness? How does one attain the desired emotion in a treatment? Am I going to consciously embarrass myself by becoming a "hair whisperer"? Will I merely be considered a weird woman who talks to her mustache?

How come Gabriel supports the guide but still doesn't completely support the concept?

Do I have to provide photographic proof that it works? Will there be questions I can't answer? Will people like the theory? How many will actually try the method? How will I respond if people ask me why I didn't treat my mustache daily? Did I not want to? I was more interested in researching the issue. I enjoyed the idea of energetic hair removal more than achieving hairless skin.

Do we sometimes wish to help others attain happiness more than we desire to contain it ourselves? I was inundated with questions and uncertainties but, at the end of the day, I continued to type my words simply because I enjoyed doing it.

Celebrity Hair

It was evening; Gabriel had just come home from work, and I had a hot drink in my hand.

"I sent you a link to an article that was published today about a model called Morgan Mikenas, a fitness coach who stopped removing her hair,"[13] said Gabriel, going to the fridge and taking out white cheese and hot pepper that was always part of his meal.

"I saw it, she's pretty. It must take a lot of courage to publish pictures of such hairy legs. But the first things I looked for in the pictures were her eyebrows and mustache, which she clearly shapes and removes, so it isn't that much of a big deal. It seems as though no woman completely gives up removing her facial hair."

"If you say so."

"Hang on, actually, the painter Frieda Kahlo didn't bother to do her eyebrows. She grew them and made a unibrow as a trademark of her self-portraits."

"You sometimes have to be provocative to succeed," said Gabriel, taking crackers out of the cupboard and putting the food on the table.

---

13. Ethan Gefen, "Beautiful, shapely, and hairy: the fitness blogger who didn't remove her hair for a year," ynet, 23.4.17.

"The table's a mess; can't you put cups and plates in the sink on your way to the kitchen?"

"It's not a mess; it's order within chaos," I said, aware that it wasn't okay.

I picked up the plates and wiped the table with long, straight motions.

"I read the article. She was just tired of wasting time shaving and wanted to inspire women and make them feel free to do what felt comfortable to them," I tossed the rag straight into the sink.

"Did you read the Israeli reactions to the article?" asked Gabriel as he sat down.

"There are cherry tomatoes," I said, taking them out of the fridge. I washed four tomatoes under the tap, put them into a small, green plastic bowl, and handed them to Gabriel. Sitting down to rest, I took a long sip of the warm drink. Opening the article on my smartphone, I scrolled down to read the reactions to the model's hairy legs.

"Most of the reactions express revulsion and hostility, as if the article touched on a sensitive, painful point, but there are some approving reactions. I get the idea.

The news is ridiculous, they're just making an issue out of it. Many women have decided to not remove their hair. She's a lovely woman with the gimmick of a model and a fitness coach. She's not exactly making history here."

"Isn't she?" Gabriel split open a cherry tomato in his mouth.

"I found an Israeli group of hairy women on Facebook. More accurately, they are women who have chosen to stop removing their hair and they support each other as if this were the most important struggle of their lives. They correspond with each other about the article. From what they write it seems to me they get more pain than pleasure from the hair they've decided to nurture. They are so protective of their hair and are willing to accept such scorn and rejection from society; it seems as if a woman's body hair is in danger of extinction."

"Which might be a good thing for most women."

"True," I smiled, bringing the cup to my lips. I discovered it was empty. "But maybe if hair does become extinct, it would cause the body or, perhaps, the entire world, to lose its natural balance," I joked, and Gabriel smiled. His response gave me confidence.

"Women and young girls assert that their free choice to think independently has been taken away by the media. Because of this, several famous women have been photographed with full armpit hair. I first encountered this phenomenon many years ago when I saw a photograph of Julia Roberts at the Oscars award ceremony for 'Notting Hill.' She waved, exposing her hairy armpit as she walked along the red carpet. I saw the photograph in the newspaper and didn't think much about it because it didn't seem probable. Roberts is my favorite Hollywood actress and I was certain it was fake news. I didn't believe it. I thought it was nonsense and turned the page. Only recently, with all my awareness of the issue, I again saw the picture on the internet and realized it was real."

Gabriel enjoyed a cracker with cheese.

"I read that Madonna exposed a hairy armpit when she was still in high school.

I think it's proof that armpit hair symbolizes adolescence."

Gabriel gazed at his plate.

"A few years ago, she published a photograph of herself with a really hairy armpit."

"I'm eating!" he was indignant.

"Sofia Loren also exposed a hairy armpit during the fifties," I mentioned an actress closer to his age.

He opened his eyes. "Sofia Loren?"

"And Britney Spears, Miley Cyrus, Beyoncé, Drew Barrymore, and Lady Gaga; they all resist the convention of plucking hair. And many other women across the world promote and embrace the new body standard of exposing their armpit hair in public.

"These women are so despairing and frustrated by the ritual of hair removal and the need to be permanently cleansed of hair that they have simply surrendered to the force from which it's impossible to be completely liberated. It is like Stockholm Syndrome."

"You mean developing a bond with a captor?"

"Yes, they no longer participate in the struggle and they allow their hair to grow freely. When they raise their arm high to proudly show everyone the hair, they don't notice that their arm looks like a pole as if they are humbly presenting a white flag, or more accurately, a bent flag of hair.

Maybe they haven't noticed that they've gone through a mental process. They've shifted perspective in how they relate to their body hair. But most people haven't changed their thinking, and so they cannot expect sympathy.

The women's Facebook groups all say that at first, they were disgusted by the sight of the hair, but they gradually got used to it. After a while, they fell in love with their body hair like a peacock with its feathers."

"At least a peacock has colorful feathers," Gabriel finished his meal and leaned back.

"Some women dye their armpit hair different colors; I think it looks great."

"That's very nice. Is there anything else? I'd appreciate tea and dessert."

"And some do occasionally remove their armpit hair when they go out to a public or family event and don't wish to find themselves in a storm of public pressure. Afterwards they regrow it. I find it difficult to believe. If someone told them that with the press of a button they could get rid of hair naturally, once and for all for free and be in harmony with their hair, they'd immediately toss their feminine agenda and try to see the extraordinary response of the hair."

"Don't be so sure; people don't change their minds so quickly."

"In any case, I respect everyone's path. It doesn't matter if they choose to be beautiful with or without hair."

I got up to see what the tall kitchen cupboard had to offer for dessert. I opened the doors and scanned the sweet contents: waffle cookies, Goji berries, and buckwheat biscuits.

"We have halva hair," I read aloud.

Gabriel didn't respond.

Help

We seem to have an unofficial principle of staying home, maybe because we're paying rent and it seems a pity to waste time outside the house. But this kind of thinking necessarily leads to a constant strolling among rooms to utilize time and space. However, the wedding of a friend from the Moshav where we used to live was a good reason for us to leave the house.

I didn't have anything to wear to the wedding. Finding clothes in a store is not one of my skills. And, anyway, external appearance is of secondary importance to me. Gabriel is never worried that I'll keep him waiting. A few minutes before we left, I found a dark green buttoned blouse with a fine pink hood and long black pants. That's just how it is; I wear what I have and won't apologize for it.

I knew several people at the wedding and a pleasant young couple from the Moshav invited us to sit at their table, next to the entrance door of the hall.

In the middle of the evening, Gabriel came from the direction of the dance floor with someone I didn't know, his hand on his shoulder. They walked past me. The man nodded to me, said, "hello", and left the hall with my husband. I didn't recognize him because I'd only seen him once before. After staring for a few minutes at the noisy, active dance floor, I went outside. I was curious, realizing that he was a good friend of the bridegroom.

I stood, arms folded, and observed them approaching me.

"Remember him?" Gabriel addressed me.

"I do remember you. You once spent a weekend on the Moshav with Dan."

"Talk to him," said Gabriel, and he went back inside the hall, leaving me alone in the yard with the man.

I didn't grasp what was happening.

"I remember you as well," he said.

"Remind me of your name," I asked.

"Alex."

"That's right, Alex," I smiled.

"Gabriel told me about your idea of advertising a product on the internet."

"I'm writing a guide. I remember that you work on the internet." He was considered extremely professional in the field.

"I'd be glad to help you. You know I also helped Dan advance in High Tech."

"I remember your story," I nodded to him.

The bride and groom emerged and came towards us. I pressed the bride's hand. She was a Brazilian convert who glowed with an exotic, modest appearance.

"I'm glad you came," Dan said to me.

"Mazal Tov!" I formally congratulated them.

"You know, I helped Dan get ahead when he was young," Alex said to the new bride, "we're close friends."

"It's a pleasure to meet you. Dan told me about you," she responded warmly.

"You've found a good man."

"He helped me a lot when I first started out," confirmed the groom, pressing Alex's hand firmly before continuing on his way with his bride.

"So," Alex turned to me, "I'll be glad to help you; give me your telephone number and I'll send you my digital business card with all the contact details."

"Great, thank you," I answered. This was help; exactly what I needed.

I was glad that there was someone professional who can help me distribute the guide. I believed I could trust Alex to do good work.

The next day I e-mailed him the file with the guide and a week later I tried to get his opinion through a text. He answered that he was busy and hadn't had time to review the material and that he'd read it at the first opportunity. I didn't know if he was telling the truth or whether he was trying to get out of it, but I had no choice but to wait. A week went by. He sent me a message expressing genuine enthusiasm, saying that if he'd known it was so interesting, he'd have read it sooner. He added that "the guide filled in gaps for him."

I was glad to know that I'd contributed and said I needed time to edit the file and would return it to him when I felt the guide was completely ready.

I felt that if it were possible, I'd spend the whole day writing the guide. Of course, I had the odd free hour here and there, but I was frustrated by my lack of free time for writing as well as my fatigue at night. Nonetheless, I felt a rise in spirits with every word I wrote. I took note of the page numbers as proof of my progress.

For sure, perseverance would lead me to the goal of presenting my theory to anyone interested in knowing about it.

Maybe I was getting ahead of myself. I knew I had to allow things to develop naturally without being pressured. Even if this made sense, it was still annoying. But it is vital to be able to enjoy the journey and not only the result. The beauty lies in how we see all the stages of progress because, ultimately, the result will remain constant.

My word count showed nine thousand words. It seemed like an advanced guide to me and I was proud of myself.

In parallel, I gradually made progress with my mustache treatment. I was indifferent and didn't try to make the hair stop growing all at once, not even for my guide. I understood the little girl inside of me and I didn't pressure myself to speed up the process any further.

***

"Alex hasn't answered my last text," I said.

"You said he liked it," responded Gabriel.

"Yes, he seemed enthusiastic and he got the idea quickly. He's smart and he managed to read between the lines beyond the removal of hair."

"So, what happened?"

"I don't know why people cool off so fast," I answered coldly.

The sound of an incoming text message was heard from my smartphone. I hurried to check.

"It's Alex, saying he's moved to live in Russia with his girlfriend and has taken on more projects. He's under pressure at work and can't help me after all," I told Gabriel. He looked disappointed.

"It's all for the best," I said "I'm not even certain I'm writing just a guide. I have nine thousand words and I've begun to wonder if my internet guide isn't a small book that has to grow and be published on paper with a designed cover. It should find its place on a shelf in a bookstore."

Gabriel examined my face. "Maybe he's trying to steal your idea."

"No conspiracies, please. Today I printed out the guide to see what it would look like as a book. It's thrilling to see how ideas and words from my mind have become something tangible."

Gabriel got up and went out onto the sun balcony off our bedroom that served as an evening spot for quiet conversations. Our blocked view was a wall with the windows and air-conditioners of a religious high school. Separating us was a mesh fence covered by a green bush that flowered with large orange flowers during the winter. The bush that spread along the fence had taken over, climbing onto the tree beneath our balcony and thickly covering the top, which was adjacent to the high balcony.

"What's wrong with that plant?" Gabriel noticed that the plant had wrapped itself around our clothes lines and was holding onto the black railing.

"Do you think it's just a coincidence that it's happening now after we've been living here for two years? Maybe the plant is aware of the fact that I am working on the notion of plant and hair consciousness and is trying to approach and use the opportunity because it knows that I won't harm it even though it is taking up laundry space on the lines."

I dared not touch the plant or allow my curious boys to pick the leaves from their branches. I did not even let them pick the leaves that had nowhere to hang from and which fell heavily to the balcony floor.

The rustling of brushing leaves sounded from the treetop. Gabriel and I tensed.

"I think it's the sound of mice climbing along the electricity lines.

It's not the first time I've heard rustling," I said, squinting with an effort to see movement in the darkness.

"That's because there are so many cats in the area; the mice are forced to survive at the height of the lines." Gabriel sounded worried and as it turns out, he was right.

The Mouse

I was at the Eco Park with the boys one afternoon, in the eastern neighborhood of the city when my smartphone rang. "The lovely Adele" appeared on the monitor.

"Mom, I think there's a mouse in the house," she sounded hysterical.

"What do you mean you think?"

"I saw something running like mad out of your room."

What could I do? What did she expect?

"When I get home, I'll check it out. And tell Lia to stop screaming because I can't understand a thing anyway."

"When will you come?"

"Later."

"Mom!"

"I'm on my way, breathe."

We shortened our stay in the park and went home. I went anxiously and quietly into my room, checked around our mattress that lay on the beige carpet. I checked the bathroom, the toilet, and the living room. There wasn't much I could do about it and I hoped that the mouse had decided to go out the way it had come in.

Two days later, when I opened the oven drawer to take out baking paper, I found tiny dark droppings and what appeared to be unidentifiable, crumbling orange cotton wool. It seemed that the mouse had had time to get organized and indulge in the oven drawer as its main bedroom.

Preferring not to tell the girls about the proof of the mouse's presence at home, I knew I had to wait for the right moment to catch it. I was relieved when the time came the following morning. I was in the kitchen. The girls had gone to school and I was making a typical breakfast for the little ones, consisting of an omelet, bread, and tomatoes. My attention was caught by slight scrabbling sounds coming from the oven drawer. I realized that the source of the noise could only come from the movement of the little creature and that this was the time to try and catch it. I wasn't sure there'd be another opportunity.

Gabriel loped into the kitchen and received a firm, quiet message from me that there was a mouse in the oven. I gestured to the oven drawer, hurriedly brought the low table from the living room, turned it on its side, and positioned it between the wall and the entrance door that was wide open. In this way, I blocked off the kitchen, preventing the possibility of the mouse escaping from the kitchen into the living room and bedrooms. This was the first stage. The boys, who were sitting at the kitchen table, realized that something was happening and were following me with expressions of curiosity.

"Now we have to take the oven outside with the mouse," I said. I was certain this was the wisest and most practical solution.

Gabriel thought for a moment, then said, "turn on the oven, and the mouse will come out."

I paused. In my heart, I agreed that this was the easiest, most logical, and simplest way. I should have thought of it myself. I couldn't believe I'd considered dragging a heavy oven outside while fearing the mouse would escape on the way out, and then return the oven to its place. How come I thought of something so clumsy and technical whereas Gabriel thought of harnessing the energy of heat from the oven to make the mouse come out effortlessly by itself? I was ashamed of myself and I appreciated his not saying anything. I examined Gabriel's expression and realized that he hadn't at all grasped what I'd been thinking. Without hesitating, I swiftly and determinedly turned round and switched the oven on to maximum heat. I escaped behind the wall of the low table I'd brought in. Once they'd realized that a drama was about to take place, Ethan and Tom stood beside me.

Tensely, like me, they waited for something to happen. Gabriel volunteered to remain next to the oven in the kitchen. We all waited.

The mouse apparently began to feel the spreading and increasing heat inside the oven and with an instinct for survival, escaped. It came too close to Gabriel's feet and Gabriel yelled. The mouse fled a few feet forward behind the fridge in the corner, opposite the oven. I was afraid the mouse would decide that the fridge floor would be its new refuge, but Gabriel was already hitting the side of the fridge with a broom, hinting to it to continue running. The mouse had no alternative. With the courage of Mighty Mouse, it continued its escape to the other side of the fridge, straight towards the table barrier I'd created. With impressive timing, I leaned over the table with a broom and swept the dark hairy body out through the front door. I looked at it before it disappeared around the corner. It looked behind to see what had pushed it out. It had a frightened look in its eyes. I felt sorry for it, but this was in the interest of all parties and, in any case, according to the rental agreement, we were forbidden from subletting.

I closed the door with a sigh of relief.

"There, the mouse is gone." I told the little ones. I dragged the table back into the living room. Then, out of the corner of my eye, I saw Gabriel take a long, sharp meat knife out of the drawer and stride determinedly towards the balcony. I followed him and the little ones followed me. I understood what he intended to do. Holding the branches of the climbing bush, he energetically began to cut them away.

"Actually, it's a pity to cut it away like this, but there's no alternative," he said apologetically, either to the plant or to me.

The boys and I watched his efforts. I couldn't stop myself and said, "it's impossible to claim that plants have no eyes. It sees precisely where it can grow. It wraps the thin branches and coil around the railing to create a strong, stable structure that will hold the weight of the main branch and leaves." My words were a kind of obituary over the destruction of the branches, but we couldn't have a bridge of branches for all types of infiltrators. I realized that it was ridiculous to allow plants to take over any more of our little balcony.

"Just imagine the hair on our bodies as a sort of creeper growing all over us without boundaries; we'd go out of our minds," I chuckled.

Gabriel began to throw large branches down into the yard.

"You know, the talk experiments carried out with the plants have proved that the technique also works with body hair because they are both conscious. This is the proof! There's no need to prove it in a regular manner. There is no room for doubt."

My theory seemed clear and beautiful. When I grasped the fact that I was defining the theory as "beautiful," it became more credible and correct because I'd become a minor, informal partner with scientists and physicists who had defined their theory as something beautiful. Until now, I hadn't really understood the significance.

For me, it was a magical feeling; parts of life accurately coming together, creating a new and wonderful landscape still unseen in reality because nobody had intentionally walked through it.

Since beauty is in the eye of the beholder, the problem is that a subjective feeling about a concept doesn't yet constitute conclusive proof; it merely constitutes an excellent start. Scientists require objective proof not based on opinions, gut feelings, or emotion. So, ultimately, a theory must be properly proven.

Gabriel continued to cut away the branches, a job that took longer than he thought. The task turned out to be physically arduous. Ethan and Tom watched him with admiration, as if he were no less than a superhero who was saving the family from the evil plants taking over their home. The cutting away of branches changed nothing for them; their consciousness was too young to understand and develop sensitivity and empathy for plants.

"You haven't proved it beyond a doubt. You have no before and after photographs," panted Gabriel.

I rebelled. "I don't want to put photographs of my mustache in the book. It isn't aesthetic; it's actually revolting. I don't have to prove the theory by using photographs. It frustrates me, mainly because it's stupid. I could just use any photograph of a woman's mustache, put one without mustache hair beside it, and write that it was proof. If anything, I should photograph the hair follicles with a Trichoscope. It's the only way to prove it. And you have to remember that skeptics will have what to say no matter what."

"People won't be in a hurry to believe you."

"So what. I'm doing the work." Later that day, I sent my manuscript to three large publishing houses.

Alone?

A pleasant breeze welcomed me as I went out onto the balcony. I sat on the narrow concrete bench next to the railing. Gabriel was removing the remainder of the slender branches that were still attached to the railing but were severed from the plant.

"What an operation we had here this morning," I said.

"We must make sure the mice will have no further way in," said Gabriel with severity.

"Yes," I agreed, "however, this afternoon we had a guest of a different kind."

"What now?"

"Ethan apparently liked the idea of an animal at home and used chicken scraps to coax a stray cat into the building and up to our door."

"He likes cats. Shall we adopt one?" Suggested Gabriel.

"No way," I protested, "I don't want cat hairs all over the house."

"He really loves cats."

"He loves them? He has no idea of how to behave with them. He strokes the cat and pulls its tail even though I told him he mustn't and that the cat doesn't like it."

"It has to be explained to him again and again until he understands."

"It takes time to develop sensitivity. The problem is that in the meantime it could be at the cat's expense," I responded.

I thought to myself that it was time Gabriel read the guide I'd written, so I wouldn't have to constantly explain different parts of the concept of hair removal.

"You have to read the guide I wrote," I said as if this were the subject of our conversation.

"I can't read a guide about hair."

"But you haven't read what I've written."

"I can't read spiritual material that isn't biblical."

"That's an excuse. You read the book *Conversations with God*[14] that I brought from the library."

"That's something else."

"It doesn't matter, I'm asking you to take an interest in your wife," I said, pointing at myself.

Gabriel gave me a tender look. "Okay, I'll read it."

I floated enthusiastically towards the room and took the printed manuscript out of my closet.

Gabriel went into the room and fell belly down onto the bed. In front of him, I placed the white pages that were reflected in his glasses. Gabriel tends to read aloud, even if we are both looking at the text together. Perhaps this comes from reading the news to listeners when he worked abroad as a broadcaster for a local Jewish radio station.

He read the preface to the guide in that deep bass voice of his that I love.

---

14. *Conversations with God: An Uncommon Dialogue*, Book 1, by Neale Donald Walsch. Translation: Idit Shorer, 1997, Opus Press, Tel Aviv.

"If any process hurts consistently, you should try another approach. Any person who encounters a great problem without resolving it over time should discard his basic assumptions and the methods he used to resolve the problem, and find a creative alternative which will lead him to a new approach and way of thinking."

Gabriel glanced at some of the other papers in the guide and returned to where he'd been reading before:

"The guide to hair removal by means of energy is different from everything we know today. It will bring hope to anyone who believes he is doomed to tear his hair out for the rest of his life, with recurring attempts to remove unnecessary body hair." Gabriel began to show signs of distress. He skipped pages and read another paragraph with a swift murmur, and then went on to the next page.

"Okay, I get it," Gabriel said, putting the pages aside.

I was annoyed. "Hey, you've only just started."

"I can't read all that."

I was irritated. "You don't have to read the entire guide in one evening."

He got up and the pages scattered slightly.

"It has all sorts of interesting details," I insisted.

"I get it. Sorry, I can't read a guide on hair," he said firmly and left the room, leaving a void behind him.

I was left alone with the abandoned guide.

So he can't cope with hair. I'm aware that he is revolted by any hair not attached to its follicle and by the sight of a hair in the bathroom sink. It repels him just like any other person, maybe more, but I'd written something he should read because he is the person closest to me. He should try and understand what I'm talking about.

Is it too much to ask? Do I expect too much? Doesn't he understand how important it is to me?

I went to the door and glanced out towards the short, deserted passage. Torn and full of doubt, I leaned against the doorway.

Why was I engaged with the issue of irritating, ugly, and revolting hair? I quickly defended myself: I didn't consciously choose it, it just happened.

Why did it happen to me? I didn't ask for it; clearly there was a mistaken body address when this "enlightenment" was delivered upon me. Is it my job to distribute the theory?

Maybe I'm deluded?

I was angry with myself. I didn't want anything more; just peace and quiet.

I examined the pile of paper. For a moment, I wanted to be a drama queen. I wanted to toss the papers into the air and say to hell with them; this would be appropriate for information that was unimportant and had no value. However, I'm usually a reserved type. What was I supposed to do? I don't have to continue if I don't want to. After all, no one is forcing me to. But if I don't pass on the idea, someone else will probably do so in the future.

But does that really matter? The main question is whether I would regret it, and if I could forget the whole thing. Dear God! I'd already sent the guide to publishers.

I didn't know if I had the strength to cope with such a different, revolutionary message which would probably bring with it the need for proof and considerable explanation of something that to me appeared simple.

I looked down and my heart grew dense and heavy. I felt my energy draining. I was fading, about to collapse into myself. I was on the verge of a massive implosion that would leave a black hole sucking all things into it, even light, and everything inside it would be lost forever.

Schrödinger's Cat

Gabriel and I didn't talk about what had happened. I didn't even talk to myself about what I had written. I was on a mental break from the energetic removal of hair. In any case, I thought, it was now up to the publishers. I was in waiting mode.

In the meantime, we had a constant guest. I'd almost gotten used to Lucky the cat and I bought it a large bag of cat food.

Ethan sensed whenever Lucky was behind the entrance door. He'd open it and the cat would slink inside and go straight to its saucer of grainy food in the corner near the door. Ethan stroked it.

"Don't disturb the cat when it's eating," I tried to guide him. My words were of no interest to him.

The cat ate a little and then turned to be petted by Ethan. "Don't pick it up, you're supposed to bend down to it," I tried to offer a little more guidance. After a few seconds of affection, the cat escaped from Ethan's grasp and Ethan chased it to the closed balcony off the living room. Tom followed in pursuit. They bent down to caress it but Ethan wanted the cat for himself.

He insisted on picking up the cat again. Tom imitated his brother and held a large, furry, toy dog. It was black and white with a pink tongue.

He approached Ethan, waving the dog from side to side as if it were real. Lucky the cat opened its eyes in alarm and tried to escape from Ethan's arms but this time he held it firmly. Lucky began to squirm, and then scratched Ethan behind his ear.

"No!" I shouted, but it was too late. Ethan shrieked with pain. I was terrified. Opening the door I shouted, "get out!" The cat needed no further words of encouragement and tore out.

Gabriel came running from the room. "What happened?" His voice was anxious.

"The cat scratched Ethan because of the toy dog," I hurriedly answered, going to Ethan to see what had happened. Ethan, his eyes closed, continued to shriek, waving his hand next to the injured ear. Blood dripped onto his neck. Gabriel gently examined his ear.

"Good God," he groaned, "it's torn his ear."

"Torn his ear?" I couldn't absorb what had happened.

"Get the iodine," Gabriel ordered, forcing me to function. Trembling, I went to the kitchen.

"He's bleeding a lot," called Gabriel, taking Ethan to the bathroom to wash the wound.

Tom stood in the living room, looking at me with incredulity.

"Damn cat," I muttered, quick to tell him: "you can't play with a stray cat." I found the iodine in the medicine basket.

In the bathroom, Gabriel washed Ethan behind his ear.

"How severe is it?' I asked anxiously.
"The scratch is quite deep."
"And if the cat is sick?"
"We'll find out."

***

The girls came home that afternoon, throwing their bags as usual onto the living room floor. They then realized that Ethan was sitting motionless on the sofa.

"What's wrong with him?" asked Adele.

I created order. "Take your bags to your room. Lucky scratched Ethan."

"I told you not to bring that cat home," said Lia.

"It doesn't matter now; we've learned the hard way," I answered.

"Won't we see it here again?" she continued to ask, a tone of reproach accompanying her words.

"Not a chance," I answered shortly. She went over to Ethan to see the wound up close.

"There's Spaghetti Bolognaise," I invited everyone to calm down at lunch.

"Mom, a fork," Ethan asked.

"I always said a dog would be better," said Lia, taking the forks out of the drawer.

"I love cats," Ethan insisted.

"You love them too much," Lia answered severely.

"I'd never bring that cat into the house," said Adele.

"If it were up to me, I'd have thrown it out a long time ago," said Lia.

"Stop it," Ethan said angrily.

"We can put the cat inside Schrödinger's box," I suggested peaceably, trying to calm the storm around the table.

"What's Schrödinger?" asked Adele.

"Who is he," I corrected her, continuing, "he's a scientist who performed a mental experiment with a cat."

"Your physics?"

"Yes, 'my' physics. It was a famous mental experiment that included a cat inside a box with a radioactive device that could kill it."

"What's special about that?"

"Dr. Schrödinger was a physicist, one of the developers of Quantum Theory. He suggested examining the strange behavior of tiny particles to see how they behave on a large scale in a cat."

"I love little cats." Ethan's comment didn't surprise us.

"The only cat I love is the cat you drew in high school," said Lia. She was referring to a framed picture hanging on the wall of the girls' bedroom.

"Anyway," I continued, "the tiny particles of matter were measured in a lab and scientists discovered that they can be in superposition, meaning two possible states simultaneously. Dr. Schrödinger tried to measure what would happen to a cat in our familiar world and if a cat can be in a state of superposition."

"Supercat," cheered Ethan, and Tom laughed, his mouth full of spaghetti.

"Why a cat?" Lia didn't like the choice.

"Maybe because of the belief they have nine lives, but it's an experiment that takes place only in the mind. Dr.

Schrödinger received the Nobel Prize," I emphasized, in order to arouse their curiosity.

"In the experiment, a cat is placed in a sealed box that also contains radioactive material, which has a fifty percent chance of breaking down during the experiment. If the material breaks down, poison is released that can lead to the cat's death. But if radioactive material doesn't break down, the cat will remain alive. The question is..." I paused for a moment to increase the tension, "what is the state of the cat while the box is closed?"

"Dead," determined Adele happily and Lia nodded in agreement to the death sentence.

"It isn't dead," protested Ethan.

"The answer is that the cat in the box is in a state of superposition. Meaning, the cat is both alive and dead. Neither alive nor dead, the possibilities exist simultaneously."

"Mom, enjoy your physics," Adele gave up the complicated thought.

I completed what I was saying. "Ultimately, the certainty of a cat's life or death depends only on what we see when we open the box. According to Quantum Physics, the very participation in the experiment affects the physical measurement carried out in it and its results. This is because some of the measuring instruments are the scientists themselves and they affect the state of the phenomenon they are measuring. This means that whoever is carrying out the experiment receives results according to what he expects and believes will happen."

"How does that help us with Lucky?" Lia was still looking for revenge.

"It doesn't. The situation already happened; the cat scratched Ethan. Maybe it wouldn't have happened in a parallel world. Maybe we wouldn't have bought a furry dog or maybe we'd be living somewhere else."

"So, it's just annoying," Lia definitely did not enjoy conceptual theory.

"No, it isn't. I was also thinking about a similar theoretical experiment on a different level. Instead of a theoretical experiment focusing on the possibilities of the life or death of a cat, my experiment proposes a focus on the state of a cat's hair. It is an imaginary experiment that doesn't require lab equipment. A cat is in a box with a sophisticated laser device from the future, which causes its fur to fall out and stop growing. There is a fifty percent chance that the device will be activated and that the cat will be found without fur. What is the cat's state while it is in the closed box?"

Now it was easy.

"A cat with and without fur," said Adele indifferently in order to please me.

I smiled with pleasure. "Exactly. Only when the box is opened will there be a collapse of one of the possible states of the cat with or without fur."

"This has to do with the removal of hair, right?" Adele really got it.

"Yes, obviously. In the depths of the hair cells are super-states in which hair grows and stops growing; this is my claim. We can choose the state of hair cells."

"Mom, you also deserve to win the Nobel Prize," declared Lia.

"Thank you. It would be the Nobel Peace Prize for

resolving the age-old conflict between people and their body hair," I said.

Welcome to the world of body hair cell possibility. There are worlds of intelligent electrons with attention deficit disorder that jump out of place all the time and behave distractedly and indecisively. In the inner life of the hair cell, all situations exist: a hair grows and a hair stops growing, there is a flicker of two pictures one inside the other: hair – no hair, hair – no hair. The possibilities exist one beside the other and they possess their own internal logic.

There is no dimension of time or space. Electrons can appear and disappear, affecting other electrons.

Discussions about theoretical physics excites me. I know for certain that there is beauty and wisdom in the universe that I cannot ignore. It is irreversible knowledge that one can talk to hair and cause it to stop growing. Maybe I should acknowledge that I have more of a relationship with my body hair than feminists do. They are so proud of not removing hair. In contrast, I have developed a respect for intelligent hair, over and above the fact that it is part of my body. This in no way contradicts the fact that I don't think body hair is aesthetic, and I have no interest in changing my attitude and perception of its beauty.

I no longer felt anger or resentment towards Gabriel. I didn't feel a need to squeeze out any approval of my theory or my writing from him. I'd already found the approval within myself.

Joy that Works

I had to admit to myself that talking to mustache hair is not a task I particularly enjoy. I don't do energy treatment because I want to, but rather I do it because I need the treatment to work and I know that it can. I wondered if I should change my approach. Maybe I should approach treatment from a feeling of joy. I wasn't sure if this would actually help me to get rid of hair more successfully, but I remembered the sentence: "This joy is ... Life Itself, expressing at the highest vibration. It is supra-consciousness. It is at this level of vibration that creation occurs."[15]

The electromagnetic power of the beating heart inside us becomes strongest when we are joyful.

But is it joy alone that activates it? Does being joyful do the work? Is there no need to supervise? Demand? Get angry?

I stood in front of the mirror. It was almost entirely white from a layer of dried droplets. I sprayed the mirror and dried it with absorbent paper. It left tiny marks. I patiently wiped the mirror clean, until I could see the clear reflection of my serious image.

---

15. *Conversations with God, An Uncommon Dialogue*, Book 1, by Neale Donald Walsch. Translation: Idit Shorer, 1997, Opus Press, Tel Aviv.

I closed my eyes. I imagined my upper lip perfectly cleansed from hair. I thought to myself that this is how it would always be. I was a little excited by the thought of seeing a hair-free upper lip. I felt myself smiling. I devoted about ten seconds to this vision as there was a limit to the amount of joy I was able to experience. Opening my eyes, I began to describe to my hair what I was imagining.

"You've stopped growing." – I generated a positive feeling.
"You've stopped growing." – This was good communication.
"You've stopped growing." – I became slightly skeptical.
"You've stopped growing." – Was I joyful enough?
"You've stopped growing." – I tried to release fireworks from my heart.
"You've stopped growing." – I focused on the imagination.
"You've stopped growing." – I didn't take control.
"You've stopped growing." – I transmitted joy.
"You've stopped growing." – The hair cells were affected.
"You've stopped growing." – The hair's energy was changing.
"You've stopped growing." – The strands of hairs were slowing their vibration.

I believed in the energy of joy, but the little girl inside me wasn't totally convinced. Nonetheless, the talking process became far more pleasant. The irritable commands of activating force were replaced by a feeling of relief and inner power. I felt a more comfortable sense of cooperation.

Finally, I thanked the hair follicles. Gratitude sealed the feeling of joy inside me, no matter how faint it was.

I believed the work was done without delay, and I was free to continue my occupations, knowing that I'd left instructions in the hands of a team with the highest expertise and most classified inner knowledge; a team of messenger particles that knew how to implement its task to the best of its ability and my satisfaction.

Once too Often

"Mom, come and do my mustache," Adele called, her voice echoing from the bathroom.

"Later, I'm with the kids." We were huddled over Sammy the Firefighter - a memory game.

"But in the evening you say there isn't enough light and days go by," she said reasonably.

Leaving the boys in the living room, hoping they wouldn't scatter the playing cards, I hurried off towards her. I glanced through the door. She was examining her face in the mirror. I went into the bathroom.

"If you'd pluck with thread as I do, it would be better for you, and you wouldn't be dependent on anyone else. You're lucky I do it for you. When I was your age, my friends at boarding school would pluck my mustache with thread and I was embarrassed when they came into my personal space."

"I don't know how to do it," she hadn't even tried.

"It was hard for me too at first. I'd twist the thread in the air above my upper lip without plucking a single hair. It took time to learn to do it by myself. I'd try and despair, and try again and despair. I despaired quite a few times until I succeeded," I lectured her on perseverance.

"I don't like to use threads. It hurts too much and leaves red marks."

"How many methods of hair removal do you know?" I distracted her.

"For the mustache?"

"Sure, let's say the mustache."

"Don't know, about three: thread, wax, and tweezing."

"Out of all the possibilities, could there be one ultimate, correct, logical and natural method?" I was edging towards a particular answer.

"Could there be only one more method of removing hair that no one except you knows about? And just by chance, it is weird?" Adele teased me.

"It's worth your while to stop the growth of your mustache energetically." I touched her arm, "you're the future generation of hair removal. You have the option of receiving knowledge from me and doing more advanced hair removal by communicating with hair."

Defiantly, Adele held out a small strip of wax for removing facial hair that cost too much, thereby signaling that she wasn't interested in talking to hair.

"Your choice," I said and got to work. I rubbed the double strip between my hands to warm the wax, slightly melting it before use. I opened the strip to create two strips and placed one on Adele's upper lip and pulled upward. I examined the strip to see if there were any hairs. I raised the strip towards the light. There were several hairs but nonetheless the area I'd plucked wasn't completely free of hair. I replaced the strip and plucked again, once too often.

"Mom," she yelled in pain.

"Sorry."

Adele examined her face in the mirror. "I don't believe it!" she cried out.

I hadn't grasped what had happened.

"See what you've done!" Adele turned her face to me. A tiny, fine piece of skin under the left nostril had been removed. The skin had stuck to the wax strip, leaving exposed, pinkish flesh.

Shit. "Talk to your mustache," I demanded – not in good timing, "this is cold, hard, unintended proof that wax is a method that should be used only for a short period, in addition to talking to hair."

"I don't want to do abracadabra with my hair; I'm doing something else," she sobbed, with tears flowing down her cheeks.

"I'm sorry, it wasn't intended. I should have been more careful with the wax."

"What am I going to do now?" Her lips curved in misery and she went into an end of the world mode. She continued to examine the sore up close in the mirror.

"We'll go to the doctor and he'll give you an ointment," I said, trying to stay calm.

Adele walked around the house for several days with a thick layer of ointment on the sore. Fortunately, it soon healed.

Children Make You Grow

My father, may he rest in peace, died when I was pregnant with little Tom. The children and I occasionally visit my childhood home, which was also the landscape of the girls' childhood. My sister-in-law, who is two months younger than I am, still lived there. I knocked on the white door and we waited for an invitation to enter. When the invitation didn't come, I knocked again and went inside. Hannah came out of her room to welcome us. She was glad to see us. "Hi, what's up?"

"All is well, thank God." We hugged.

"Adele, what happened under your nose?" Asked Hannah at the sight of the white ointment. Bespectacled Ruth stood next to her mother with a curious expression.

"Just a sore," Adele dismissed the issue. She didn't want to expand on it and so I answered for her, "I was waxing her mustache and took off a piece of skin, but it's healing very well."

"Mom, that's enough!" Adele was embarrassed.

"You don't say! Wax warmed in the microwave?" Hannah was interested.

"No, we used ready strips of wax."

"Don't use them. Use wax that comes in aluminum wrapping. Don't you thread her mustache?"

"She's worse than you are, it's a nightmare removing her mustache with thread."

"Yes, pain tolerance in this family isn't exactly our strong suit," she laughed understandingly.

Ruth, Adele, and Lia were talking in the living room and Ethan and Tom began to play with their cousin, Jonathan, who was their age.

I sat down on a chair in the kitchen.

"Ruth is being harassed at school because she has hairy legs," Hannah sat down opposite me on a revolving chair.

"This is prevalent among girls her age. What do they say to her?"

"They say that she's a 'hairy monkey.' I waxed her several times but now I let her shave."

"This generation is maturing fast."

"Yes, we're even considering laser treatments for her."

"But she's only ten." I looked at her. She was in the living room with the whole gang.

"Yes, believe it or not, there's a beauty counselor especially for little girls who want to do laser treatments. They even offer laser treatment to five-year-olds. What do you have to say to that?"

"I'd say it's a tough situation. What does Ruth have to say about it? Does she also want to do laser?"

"Yes, very much, obviously."

"It'll probably hurt her."

"We're still thinking about it and forming an opinion.

Then we'll see. In the meantime, she uses a razor. What else can we do," she concluded.

"Well, there is something," I said.

"What?"

"You asked me to lend you my book *The Power of Your Subconscious Mind.*"[16]

"Yes, what's the connection?"

"If you understand the book, you can find the solution there."

I enjoyed being incomprehensible.

"Well, really, what are you talking about?"

"There's a way to get rid of hair," I felt like a magician pulling a rabbit out of a hat, "in a way that is spiritual."

"How?" Her tone was totally skeptical.

"All you have to do is ask your hair to stop growing," I said.

"Only you could say such weird things," she responded.

The rabbit I'd pulled out seemed like an alien to her. "I can explain," I said.

I knew I had to convey my theory. Reflecting on Ruth, I thought it would be interesting to simplify the theory for children.

"Call Ruth and I'll explain it to both of you. Maybe it will persuade you to reconsider hair removal by laser."

"Ruth, come here," called Hannah.

Ruth got up and asked impatiently what we were up to.

"Your Mom has told me that you're being harassed at school because of the hair on your legs," I was open about the issue.

---

16. The Power of Your Subconscious Mind, Joseph Murphy, translation: Leora Carmeli, Or-Am Publishing House, 2000.

"Yes..." She tried to understand what was going on and gave her mother a dissatisfied look.

"Do you know why girls remove their hair?" I tried to gain her attention.

"Because it's ugly," she said unequivocally.

"Maybe because we enjoy abusing ourselves; maybe we are completely mad," I teased her a little, but she seemed confused. She didn't know what I wanted from her.

"Everyone wants to be beautiful, it's a natural desire. We want to be free of hair and we don't want to look like a little furry monkey." I hoped I wasn't adding insult to injury but I did manage to interest her a bit because she smiled slightly. This was my opportunity to try and explain the theory in a way that was age-friendly.

"I have a great story for you, would you like to hear it?"

"What's the story about?" She looked at her cousins who were still absorbed in the computer, watching the clip of an American singer in a white hat, sun-glasses, and a pink jacket who was singing and dancing at the head of a group of men in the street.

"A story that will explain how to remove hair another way."

"A long story?"

"An interesting story."

She fell silent, my signal to begin.

"Fifty years ago, there was a man called Cleve Backster, an expert on police polygraph instruments."

"What's a polygraph?" Ruth sat down beside her mother.

"A polygraph is a lie detector that measures physiological responses. When a person takes a polygraph test, four sensors are attached to him and detectors help the machine to draw the exact emotional response of a person on a graph with a special needle. There is also a questioner who asks the person connected to the polygraph machine various questions. The person has emotional responses to the questions and the questioner knows if he is lying or not by the measurements the machine makes on the paper."

"How does he know?" Asked Ruth. I remembered that she wanted to be a detective when she grew up.

"When we tell the truth, our heart is calm. We are sure of what we are saying; there's no inner tension. But if the questioner asks questions that the person does not want to answer truthfully, and the person is lying or telling half the truth, then his heart starts to beat more quickly and strongly. Most people cannot control the activity of their heart or make it beat calmly, although there are some who, with practice, can do it." I had to remember that I was talking to a little girl and I didn't want to burden her with complicated information.

"One day, Backster decided to amuse himself by attaching the polygraph to the leaf of a plant to see if it aroused some response while he watered it," I continued.

Ruth was attentive.

"Backster identified an interesting response from the plant: as if it was excited by the water it received, and he decided to try and get a stronger response from the plant. Backster knew that in order to get a stronger response he had to take an extreme stand and threaten the plant.

"He dipped the leaves of the plant in hot coffee and there was no response. Then he decided to do something even more extreme: burn the leaves. Backster thought he'd bring matches from the room next door and, the moment he thought about it, quick and sharp drops and rises were recorded on the paper. The plant was agitated and perhaps afraid. Backster was astounded. Had the plant read his mind?"

Ruth's eyebrows were raised in wonder. "Can a plant read minds?"

"He went to fetch the matches and when he returned there was another rise recorded on the graph. If he hesitated or had reservations about burning the plant, the responses from the lie detectors would not have been so sharp. When he pretended like he was intending to burn the leaves, there was no response. The plant knew how to distinguish between real sensations and lies," I emphasized the end of the sentence.

"And then what?"

"He thoroughly researched the phenomenon. He learned plants..."

"So can plants hear our thoughts?" she asked again.

"Yes, they are capable of sensing our thoughts."

"How?"

"Yes, how?" Hannah joined in.

"I don't really know how, and I don't think that anyone has managed to understand it to this day, but Backster maintains that it is our five senses that prevent us from seeing and communicating better. It is apparently related to the fact that plants have a sensitivity and connection to the universal energy field. These channels are open and unlimited. Plants are very developed; they communicate with each other and they even know, from a distance of thousands of kilometers, what is going on with people to whom they are emotionally attached. Isn't it fantastic?"

"So, what's it got to do with hair?" Asked Ruth.

"A lot," I hurried to answer, "because they discovered that plants respond to people's thoughts; they experimented by speaking hurtfully to plants and it turns out that this affects them. Negative words make them wither and dry."

"Really? That's a pity. But what does that have to do with hair?" asked Ruth again.

I glanced at Hannah who was swinging from side to side on the revolving chair and was waiting for me to speak.

"The human body is a reflection; a small scale of everything in the world. The smooth hairless palm is like a dry desert.

A forest is like the hair on the head. Grass is like the hair on your legs. In addition, a similar consciousness in plants exists in the cells of your hair.

So you can talk to the hair on your legs because they hear and understand. You can tell them you want them to stop growing."

Ruth seemed to freeze. "I'm going to the computer," she said, getting up and hurrying as far away as possible, about three meters from us.

"It must have been too much for her," I said hesitantly to Hanna.

"Nonsense, she's tough." Hannah wanted to soothe me.

"Like nature, women are different from men. It is reflected in experiments as well. Even Charles Darwin's great-granddaughter spoke to tomatoes, which developed better than those that weren't spoken to. I watched videos and saw that when women spoke to an apple or to rice, they did it gently and sensitively, unlike one man I saw in an amusing but extreme video by a standup artist called Ron Babcock who talks to potted plants. You must see it. I watched it at least ten times. It's crude but very funny."

Hannah likes dark humor.

"What does he do?" She was also curious.

"He creates a warm loving relationship with one plant and really nurtures its ego as if he were its godfather. In contrast, he relates with hostility and aggression to another plant. He verbally bullies it, creating plant family dramas. It's funny, despite knowing that it is deliberate emotional abuse of the plant. I tell you, it hurt me to see the plant he abused wither up and become dry and sad. You have to see it."

I looked at the table. I expected to see my smartphone next to me.

"Call me," I asked.

Hanna opened her phone cover and dialed. We looked around until we heard my ringtone – the opening song of the series *The Big Bang*.

My smartphone was next to the boys. They were playing on the floor with a tractor and a large crane. I removed the smartphone before they took an interest in it and wrote in the search on YouTube, *plant talk. I* gave it to Hannah so she could watch the video.

I sat back in my chair. The girls were absorbed in the screen, huddled in front of the computer.

Hannah laughed aloud and Ruth got up and made her way to the kitchen, wondering what was interesting to her mother on the smartphone. Maybe she was still thinking about the things I'd told her.

"Ruth, do you know who else talks to plants?"

"Who?" She responded with an obvious lack of interest, turning her back to me and opening the fridge door.

"A real prince in London."

"William?" Hannah raised her head, "how incredible that the plant withered."

"Not Prince William; his father, Prince Charles," I said, "he already realized it was good to talk to them during the eighties."

"A prince who talks to plants?" Ruth giggled as she continued to inspect the contents of the fridge.

"A seventy-year-old prince," I winked at Hannah and turned to Ruth.

"He said it was very important to talk to plants, because he noticed that they respond. And I say it is essential to talk to the hair on your legs because it bothers you. Tell them what you want. You'll see, it will respond to you."

"Yeah, right. And it'll answer me?" Feeling despair from the fridge, she slammed the door shut, turning to open the snack cabinet.

"It won't talk to you in words, but it will respond through action. Your hair is part of you and you can simply tell it to stop growing. It's your right."

"You think so? The children will bother me even more." She took out a packet of biscuits and turned around.

"Why would they bother you? You don't have to tell anyone exactly what you're doing."

She seemed hesitant, but her eyes had a renewed spark of interest.

"Talk to your hair in the past tense; tell it that it has already stopped growing."

"How did it stop?"

Hannah intervened, "Don't make it difficult for her. She can tell it to stop growing and that's it. It works in any case, doesn't it? Just like the video."

"I'm not making it difficult for her. She's still a little girl and kids are great with imaginary games. It's perfect for her."

"It is not necessary," determined Hannah.

"I'm not sure I want to do it," said Ruth.

"Take as much time as you would like to think about it," I said.

She took several biscuits and went into the living room.

"Want to come with me to a standup show?" I asked Hannah.

"Since when do you go to stand up shows?"

"It's a new show that makes fun of people who live a radical, spiritual life; want to come?"

"I don't understand, what exactly is it about?"

"Remember Bella, my friend from the Moshav? She's a member of the Peleh Club in Tel Aviv. They have all kinds of events for spiritual people. I saw on Facebook that she intends to go to the performance of two characters who were busy looking for their true selves through spirituality and found deep meanings in everything. They realized they were in too deep and decided to make fun of the whole thing. The performance is full of expressions like 'consciousness,' 'frequency,' and 'mantra.' It's called

Enlightened Ltd. and should be great. It's their premiere performance. I really want to go, and maybe I'll see Bella on the way."

"Sounds good. Can Ron come too?" Ron is my elder brother. He despises that kind of spirituality.

"I don't think Gabriel will want to go, so I won't even bother asking him. Apart from that, he's working at the store on Saturday night."

"Great, so it'll be just the two of us."

"Good. The performance starts at eight thirty, so we'll have time to get organized and arrive without pressure," I said.

"We haven't been out together in years," Hannah smiled.

"Yes, we spent most of our leisure time going to the Superpharm to buy an enormous number of diapers on sale."

Difficult Hair

Lia regarded herself with satisfaction in the mirror opposite the dining table.

"My hair is really long."

"It really does look long. You have it up all the time so it's hard to see the length."

She looked different to me. To my noticing eye, her hair looked smoother. Lia has puffy, dense, and curly hair. She'd frequently asked with tears of resentment and frustration why she was the only one in the family with straw-like puffy hair.

"Have you done something to your hair?" I asked.

"No."

"Your hair looks straighter. Have you put cream on it?"

"I haven't put anything on it," she was annoyed.

"It looks different. Have you been talking to it?"

"Yes," she responded, embarrassed, "several times."

"Well, it certainly looks different." I could hardly believe my eyes. "Incredible. If you continue, I'll include you in The Guide. But talk to it every day."

"The chestnut color is gone."

"True, you used to have chestnut colored hair."

"It's because Grandma straightened my hair years ago. The straightening burned my hair and it darkened."

"Is it connected?"

"Yes. When I'm done telling my hair to grow straight, I'll talk to it about going chestnut like it used to be."

"Okay," I laughed.

"Do you promise that my hair will be completely as straight as it is after it's been straightened?"

"Of course, I promise." I completely believed in the theory.

"Promise?"

"I promise that it should work."

"I saw Jesse from 'Full House' talking to his hair in front of the mirror, commanding it to be tidy. It was the seventh season, third episode, did you see it?" Lia asked enthusiastically.

"Don't remember. It's an old series. It's nice that you know exactly which season and which episode." I wasn't pleased about the long hours she spent in front of her smartphone screen.

"Watch it, it's absolutely up your street."

"At least Jesse inspired you; when I told you to talk to your hair, you weren't interested."

"He's cute." Putting her hand on her heart, Lia had the look of someone in love.

Enlightened Ltd

Tall street lights shone, and cars filled the road. I was contemplative.

I wondered how I could expect people to talk to their hair if they weren't connected to their spirituality; it might seem insane to them or impossible, even in their imagination.

Hannah was ready when I arrived to pick her up for the performance in Tel Aviv.

"Turn on Waze and type in Peleh Club," I requested.

She turned on her smartphone. I began driving and, as if talking to myself I said: "At the performance there will be people with different ways of perceiving spiritual experience."

"Is that a problem?"

"I'm not often exposed to different life approaches."

"Such as?"

"Bella, for instance, has treated people through Sound Healing Therapy for a long time. She uses Tibetan bowls, creating sound vibrations that are beneficial for the body."

"Is that alternative medicine?"

"A type of alternative medicine…she also leads sacred singing circles."

"And that's alternative singing?"

I laughed. "As I understand it, sacred singing is a meeting of unity and love among people, which is expressed through song, music, and prayer."

"Have you participated in a circle like that?"

"No. I left the Moshav just as Bella was starting her sacred singing circle. She once invited me to a circle but I didn't go. I hope she isn't mad at me. I trust spiritual people not to get mad and not let their negative feelings fester inside. Maybe I should have gone. Maybe I should open up more to various things."

We reached the address twenty minutes later.

We were sure we'd come to the right place, but found ourselves disconcertedly facing the white wall of a rough sealed off house without any sign of an entrance. We didn't understand the riddle or the joke. What were we supposed to do in front of a wall?

We saw a young man in a simple, white cotton T-shirt standing under a streetlamp. He was standing alone with his back to us and we weren't sure what he was doing there. Was he also looking for the entrance? We asked him – because there was no one else to ask – if he knew the location of the Pele Club. He explained that we had to go around the left side of the building because the entrance was on the other side. Back we went and we entered a short, dark, and narrow alleyway. We discovered an industrial zone and garage opposite the entrance to the club. Several people were sitting in the dark to the left of the narrow alley and a strange smell of cigarette smoke met us. The entrance door to the club was locked and we preferred to wait outside the gate, opposite the garage, and pass the time in conversation between sisters-in-law.

As I became curious to know what the place looked like inside, the door was opened by a smiling young man. We were among the first to enter. I scanned the place: on my right was a long, narrow kitchen that was clean and tidy and loaded with dishes. To my left was a small corner for hot drinks, offering cocoa and herbal teas. On the opposite side was a long, striking, red curtain. It covered a large arched opening that led, I assumed, to the main performance hall. We turned right towards a medium sized room at the center of which were two sofas and a table. White plastic chairs were placed on top of each other in two piles. I liked the furniture: a simple wooden bookcase holding books on spirituality.

I told Hannah I was going to the restroom. I wanted to see the design. The walls of the restroom were covered in a large painting of an aquarium. The toilet seat was transparent plastic with a painting of a dolphin. Small brown and gray stones were scattered in the sink. For a moment, I thought we had to rub our hands on the stones under the stream of water, but fortunately I noticed a blue bottle of liquid hand soap. I washed my hands, just for the pleasure of it. The soap smelled of the sea.

Hannah had already sat down on a chair, and another one was waiting for me. The flow of people increased. I observed them, and they seemed normal.

Although a little late, the large curtain finally opened and we hurried inside. I liked the main room; it was large, open and spacious. A tall tree that looked real stood to one side, seeming to grow out of the floor tiles while supporting the ceiling with its thick palm-like branches. On the floor were colorful carpets and black seating cushions with a back support.

Hannah and I looked for somewhere comfortable for women with rigid muscles who had never done yoga before or had trouble sitting on the floor in meditation for long periods of time. To our restrained relief, we saw three sofas against the right-hand wall. We exchanged looks. Clearly, this was the place for us. We settled back in abundant comfort. After a few minutes of waiting, once the audience had finally sat down, the performance began.

SCENE 1

A lovely blond actress in a long white Boho Chic dress sat down at a small table on which was a bottle of water and two empty glasses.

An actor with a spiky haircut entered. "Hi, I'm Grass." He held out his hand.

"I'm Feather, glad to meet you," the actress held out her hand and smiled.

"Sorry I'm late. I couldn't find a place to tether my unicorn," he apologized, half boastful.

"You have a unicorn? Wow! What type?" She asked admiringly.

"The new one, Galaxy 7S," he responded with feigned indifference.

"That's amazing," she nodded vigorously.

"Have you been waiting a long time?" Grass sat down in front of her.

"Time? What's time? The time is now," smiled Feather.

"Do you often use the app 'With all this Self-searching, I Find Myself Alone?'"

"Honestly, I do. I use it quite often." She clasped her hands. "But no one is really on my frequency."

"I understand. I'm a festival producer and never have a problem with women, but I'm looking for something real and accurate."

"Real and accurate," she agreed in a whisper, adding, "I'm a therapist. I treat with the use of the method 'Who is dumb? I'm dumb.'"

"Cool. What's that?" He leaned towards her.

"I ask my clients a question and after they answer, I ask them 'who is dumb?" and they answer, "I'm dumb!"

She demonstrated the roles of therapist and client, moving her head from side to side every time she changed roles:

"Who is dumb? I'm dumb!"

"Who is dumb? I'm dumb!"

"Who is dumb? I'm dumb!" She raised her voice in a scream, at once calming down and comfortably explaining, "they admit their stupidity in this way, and they are completely humiliated. From there one can grow." She smiled with self-satisfaction.

"That is so cool. Let's order something. Are you hungry?"

"Actually, I'm on a toxin cleansing diet, so no. But if you're hungry, go right ahead."

"Maybe some water in the meantime?" Grass was hesitant.

"Yes, water. I'm really going wild today," she giggled.

"Water, let's go wild," he smiled and poured the water. He brought the glass to his lips.

She stopped him.

"What about the blessing?" She asked in amazement.

"To life?" Grass mumbled in embarrassment, the glass in mid-air.

"Close your eyes!" she said, and noticing that he wasn't cooperating, she commanded: "Close your eyes!" She closed her eyes. She began to take long breaths. Breathing in and breathing out, she uttered with emphasis: "Thank you for the rain that fell with joy, seeping into the earth to become groundwater. Thank you to the groundwater and the rocks that enabled it to flow among them. Thank you to the worker who drew the groundwater and to all the beautiful souls who walk with me," she let out a long sigh and opened her eyes. Grass opened his eyes too and sighed deeply.

When the performance was over, the audience gave a long, standing ovation. Whistles filled the air. The actors bowed several times and were obviously happy with the success of their first performance.

Hannah and I felt no affiliation with the place, and we hurried out. Among the crowd I saw Bella. Our eyes met and we made our way to each other and hugged. I remembered how much I missed her.

"I'm going to say hi to the guys," she said, hurrying away to the actors.

Outside the club a pale moon looked down on us, willing to accompany us on our way.

"What did you think of the performance?" I asked.

"What did *you* think of the performance?" Echoed Hannah.

"Care Bears looking for meaning in the city that doesn't stop", I thought I'd found a suitable title.

"You got that right, huh!" She laughed.

"The performance was excellent. It exposed a new style of a fictional-spiritual-show that maybe stems from the search for a life of meaning, which people think they've lost. All in all, it was amusing, new and fresh. When I looked at the audience, I thought it could have been more interesting if they weren't all so soulful."

"What does it matter?"

"It matters. Some people are connected to a spiritual life, while others find it a jumble of nonsense and delusion. Here I am, writing about energetic hair removal although I don't think about the issue in this way. As far as I'm concerned, it's realistic and all about science. The concept of my theory started with science. I'm just afraid of all the skeptics who will say it's bullshit."

"Sweetheart, you don't seem to know where you're going. Of course there will be people who will say that. Prepare yourself so that you don't take it to heart. Ultimately, it took me years before I connected to spirituality through you."

"I didn't try to connect you to spirituality. When you woke up, I was there. That's all. But I'm not really afraid of being laughed at; I just don't think I want to convince people of the true power of the theory."

"What do you mean? Isn't that what you want to do?"

I stopped and faced her. "If a child in your kindergarten said you were stupid for some reason, would you get excited?"

"Yeah, right!" She grinned.

"That's how I feel. Anyone who says that energetic hair removal is nonsense, is, as I see it, a child in their understanding of this specific issue. Why should I bother with the opinions of a minor? I don't want to take to heart everything someone of little faith thinks, and I don't want to argue too much with someone who doesn't want to know."

"You need to be prepared for all kinds of reactions," she said decisively.

We left the industrial zone and continued past tall office blocks with dark, glowing windows.

Something softened inside me. "Apart from that, skepticism is a lack of faith among people who need data and scientific evidence. I can understand the skepticism, since there is no logical understanding of how energy affects matter. The problem lies in a lack of accuracy in the definition, which causes lack of understanding. Energy seems to affect matter, but the truth is that matter itself constitutes energy. Science shrieks out that our body, like the entire world, is made of energy that creates the particles. It is easier to grasp and understand that energy affects energy and thus 'matter' can absorb the influence of energy. They are at different levels. It all depends on what we want to focus on. Energy body treatments should be more logical for everyone, not only for various spiritual people like the ones we saw at the performance who are connected to their inner emotions and supposedly disconnected from reality. Enthusiastic talk about the energy in a hidden internal layer has long been the lot of Nobel Prize winning scientists who discovered through science the infinite potential of the abstract raw material known as energy. It's all a matter of open-mindedness, understanding, and perceiving the world through new concepts and ideas. We will never understand with our minds or senses the great wise energy in the depths of our body's cells which seem to contradict our senses, making us believe that our world is only tangible."

"I'll wait for your guide. I can't keep up."

"What's happening with Ruth and the laser?" I asked.

"We don't know. The whole business of hair removal is by no means a simple one, and with a little girl it is so much more complicated."

"Let's do this: I will tell you all the advantages of energy treatment and you will work out the disadvantages of all the other methods."

"Okay," Hannah nodded.

"First of all, I have to point out that treatment through energy is free."

"Very important."

"The percentage of women who shave their legs is at an all-time high. This is probably because it's the cheapest method around."

"Obviously," Hannah agreed.

"The energy treatment has a one hundred percent success rate."

"Don't exaggerate. Who else has tried to remove hair with this method apart from you?"

"Theoretically and practically this method has a one hundred percent success rate. It can't fail. One may not connect with the theory, but it is based on a natural law that doesn't change from one person to another."

"Let's assume," she seemed not to try or even want to enter a debate.

"That any place on the body can be treated," I said.

"Great!"

"Complete privacy is ensured during the treatment."

"Now you're talking!" she cheered.

"Painless," I emphasized.

"Great," said Hannah.

"It's the most advanced 'tool' in the market, and there will never be a more advanced one," I said excitedly.

"I'm in, and it's free too. Thank you."

I was satisfied. "Tell me, isn't it risky?"

"I know what you mean, I've thought about it. If we tell the hair to stop growing, would it cause the body's cells to stop growing or create some other negative reaction? First of all, the body's cells don't grow, but rather they multiply. Talking to them is innocent and unlikely to arouse a problem. The best way to feel calm is to talk specifically to the hair. For instance, 'hair, you've stopped growing,' and then the intention is specific and related to hair."

Hannah nodded.

"Hair cells are not in a state of distress or, alternatively, in a state of joy due to the energy treatment to stop the growth. The cells are experiencing daily reality. They have no long-term plans for a long life when the melanin runs out. "

"What's that?"

"The matter that gives the hair its color," I replied. "One of the most important and basic laws in the world of physics is the conservation of energy. The law determines that energy doesn't become nothing, but rather expands to take on another form. Hair is like water that turns into steam. To be accurate, with hair treatment, energy is diminished and its material structure becomes blurred. Apart from that, I even think it's healthy. Think of Ruth: the pressure she experiences from the need to remove hair all the time, the frustration when she cuts her legs while shaving, and all the other troublesome phenomena. Another point to consider is this: do you know why I think this is the perfect method?" I didn't wait for her answer, "because when I buy a product, I check to see if it contains the threesome: quality, beauty, and price. Removing hair energetically is the most natural and internal way, and it is a completely free treatment."

Hannah tried to say something, but I didn't give her the chance. I hurried to continue, "but it is great that you asked. It shows that the concept seems possible to you. Otherwise, how could it be risky if it isn't supposed to work? "

She rallied. "It's stressful. But you're right, it's easier to believe that if something bad could happen it would happen, as opposed to believing that hair will stop growing with ease and comfort."

"Murphy is long gone, and it's time that pessimism disappeared too."

"True, I'm totally with you," she exhaled.

"There's no problem with tattoos, medication, and prominent veins in the course of treatment."

"Okay, drop it." Details like that weren't relevant for her.

"You can treat yourself every day or even three times a day."

"Before or after meals?"

I ignored her teasing. "It's suitable for any skin color, pigment, or hair thickness."

"It will be interesting to see the face of the beauty consultant from the laser institute when she hears about this method." Hannah laughed.

"During the treatment, you can tan in the sun if you like."

"We don't go to the beach as much as we used to in the summer."

I couldn't stop. "It's the only method that can ensure both permanent treatment and a sense of control of the body."

"Is it for life?"

"I've been engaged in this process for quite a long time and the results remain. Theoretically, the treatment is supposed to bypass hormones. It's supposed to be a permanent hair removal treatment."

"Good, we'll try it. Listen, it's huge."

We were close to the car.

"By the way, are you coming with me?"

"Of course I'm coming with you. You're taking me home, sweetheart."

"No," I smiled, "I meant are you coming somewhere else."

"Ice-cream in Jaffa? Now?"

I opened the car with the remote and the lights switched on. "Gregg Braden is coming to Israel on the 9th of February." I felt as though he was coming personally for me.

"Who is he?" Hannah asked when we were both seated in the car.

"The coolest spiritual scientist of the century."

I turned the ignition key.

"Is it a lecture?" She put on her safety belt and I drove out of the parking place.

"He's been lecturing all over the world for years, and I wondered if he'd ever come to Israel. Now that he's coming and there's a date for his lecture, I'm hesitating for some reason. I was looking at the auditorium page to choose a seat in the hall and almost bought a ticket. Gabriel won't come with me and I don't mind going alone, but the problem is that it's on a Friday. It is a short day, and it really doesn't suit me."

"If you've waited so long, won't you go?"

"Don't know. I don't know what'll be happening in three months' time…"

I concentrated on the fact that I had another hour's journey ahead. "It is interesting that there's a distortion in time when returning home. Mostly, it seems as though the way back is shorter or rather that the time of the journey passes more quickly."

"Yes, that's true," said Hannah, "how come?"

"Time is relative; it relates to consciousness or emotion." I shrugged.

"How would I know? Am I Einstein?"

A Story

A torrent of rain fell on the balcony and a fierce wind whistled through the leaves. The weather added to my despondency. I felt empty, small, and cold.

I withdrew under the quilt in the bedroom.

The front door opened and closed, and steps approached.

"Asleep?" Gabriel whispered.

"No," I replied.

"What's wrong? Come here."

I was silent.

"What's wrong?"

I pulled the blanket away from my head. "I'm still thinking about missing Gregg Braden's lecture last week."

"But you couldn't have gone anyway because the date fell on the bar-mitzvah at the hotel and there was no way you'd have arrived on time for the event."

I hesitated with my answer. It was hard for me to say words that would establish a reality once they were said.

"I received another rejection email today from the publisher," I said with difficulty.

"It happens to most new writers; it's to be expected.

Very few receive a positive answer," Gabriel encouraged me in his way.

"The guide might not have been perfect but how come they didn't see the potential?"

"Don't despair," Gabriel said rather indifferently, turning to leave the room. Shaking myself, I jumped off the mattress. Quite suddenly, I had no intention of giving up. His presence empowered and comforted me. I knew that in order to find a solution to writing my guide, I was capable of creative thought and brainstorming with a listener.

Gabriel checked the rice on the gas in the kitchen. A burst of adrenaline spread through me and I was looking for a way to release the pressure. I took a round disposable plastic container of goji berries out of the kitchen cupboard. I scooped up a large amount and put it all in my mouth at once. It was far more than I could chew and what's more, the goji berries were rather dry. I had to chew hard and, like a delicate system of gear wheels, I felt my jaw muscles straining to work vigorously while propelling my temples and the wheels of my brain.

"Are you alright?" Gabriel lit the gas under the pot and replaced the long lighter in the oven glove hanging from a nail on the wall.

The goji berries prevented me from replying. Gabriel stirred the rice in the pot.

"I did a trivia test and it looks like I'm a genius," he said enthusiastically, waving his smartphone. I nodded to him, striving to finish what was in my mouth.

Gabriel bent over the smartphone.

"Maybe I'll write a guide, like an American quiz and,

through answering the questions, people will understand the theory," I managed to say with my mouth half full.

Gabriel scrolled through virtual pages on his smartphone.

"Maybe I'll write a story, as if the guide were already published and a bestseller. As though Oprah Winfrey interviews me and my answers convey the message."

"O-kay," said Gabriel, looking at me. I immediately recognized the pity in his eyes. He didn't really know how to help me. Clearly, my ideas were clumsy and not simple.

"It needs to be simple, which I already know, and it needs to be relatively light and flowing. Nothing new. I don't need to reinvent the wheel." I put a reasonable amount of goji berries in my mouth.

"How were things with the children today? Is Tom still hanging things on his ear?"

I nodded. "Today he walked around the house with a key ring on one ear and a small pencil behind the other."

"Maybe the child is a carpenter."

"He isn't anything of the sort. He's just a child, a baby. He doesn't talk a lot. Maybe he prefers writing…"

Gabriel filled a plate with rice.

"I know", I cried out before formulating the idea in full, "the best way to convey the theory is simply to write my story."

"Okay," Gabriel said, not understanding what all the fuss was about.

My brain kicked into overdrive.

First Haircut

My little Tom is three years old. He is at the age when, according to Kabbalistic tradition, it is customary to have the first haircut.

I came in and closed the front door behind me, leaving the boiling heat outside. I put the shopping bags down on the kitchen table. Loud voices were coming from the bedroom and I went to see what was happening. I wanted to tell Tom formally that the time had come at last for him to have a haircut. I liked the idea of no longer struggling to gather his hair into a ponytail which he insisted on undoing.

I went gladly into the bedroom, opened the door, and saw red. Tom's hair was already cut! Horror! Ethan had also had a haircut that was too short, both sides of his head were shaved with an elliptical island of hair in the middle of his head.

"You've made a Mohawk out of him?" I was stunned and ashamed. How would I go out into the street with him?

"Don't make an issue of it in front of the boy," Gabriel told me.

I tried to remain calm. "Great, Ethan. Dad cut your hair?" I smiled a forced smile.

"Yes, does it look good?" He looked up at me with his innocent eyes.

"Of course, very good, but the hair in the middle needs to be cut," I tried to convey the message gently.

"But then all the hair on his head will be too short," Gabriel protested, thereby admitting his mistake.

"There's no choice," I replied. This would be the least ugly option.

I again examined Tom's haircut. It looked as if Gabriel had used all the parts of the hair clippers, resulting in varying layers of hair. He looked like a girl. Fortunately, we were at the beginning of the summer vacation before Tom started kindergarten for the first time.

"We were planning to take Tom to Benny the barber. What's this about? Saving money?" I said resentfully in a low tone. Gabriel didn't respond. I couldn't look at my cute little boys, preferring to go to the kitchen and make them a late breakfast.

That afternoon, when Gabriel had gone to work, I mustered up the courage to clip away the hair from the middle of Ethan's head. The result was a uniform, almost bald, crew cut. He seemed to feel uncomfortable, deciding to wear a peaked cap when we went out to the barber. We drove a short distance. Even though Tom's haircut wasn't even, we felt festive. We were moved; our Tom had grown and we were parting from his childish hair. I found a parking spot in front of the barber. Luckily, no one was there. I hadn't made a prior appointment.

Benny the barber in his checked cap appeared with his usual huge smile.

"Hello, hello," he welcomed us, clapping his hands with joy.

"Hello," I smiled from the entrance to the barber shop. "We've come to repair a home haircut, which is also partially the traditional first haircut," I apologized for not coming to him in the first place.

"How nice. Tom is three years old already – a big boy who can do anything," Benny addressed me, "don't worry Mom, lots of people think cutting hair is simple and then they come to me to fix it. Believe me, I've seen more than a few terrible attempts," he soothed me, dismissing the "disaster" with a wave of the hand.

Tom looked at Benny the barber and clung to me. Ethan, on the other hand, felt more comfortable. "Mom, help me up on the chair," he asked.

"Are they both getting a haircut?" asked Benny.

"More or less," I replied, "Ethan just needs the ends done."

"Ethan you're first," called Benny, fulfilling his wish and swinging him up onto the red chair in the shape of a car. He wound a shiny black apron around him and sprayed water onto his short hair that shone from the drops. Ethan enjoyed the coolness.

"Did you take Tom to Mt. Meron for a haircut?" Benny was interested.

"Not our style," I smiled, "we celebrate with a chocolate cake from the supermarket and fireworks. It's enough."

"Great," Benny beamed and switched on the clipper.

"It looks like easy work with a clipper," I found myself

apologizing again. I sat down on an armchair next to the large mirror.

"Always come to me so they look tidy," suggested Benny as he skillfully arranged the ends of Ethan's hair around his neck and behind his ears.

The haircut didn't take very long. Soon it was Tom's turn and he was swung up into the car chair.

"You sit quietly, good for you. You're a real hero," Benny addressed him.

"Superman," murmured Tom.

"Samson the hero," I said, preferring a Jewish, less Hollywood-like hero.

"Mom, how shall I cut his hair? Buzz cut, right? Not much choice."

"Short but not too short," I requested.

"Samson the Hero whose strength lay in his hair. Incredible, huh?" Benny referred to my previous remarks.

"Yes, but if everyone was Samson the Hero, you'd have no customers," I joked.

"Wealth is a gift from God," he raised his finger.

Benny was a spiritual, broad-minded, and religious man who was always happy to share his knowledge, so I probed.

"I've noticed that men with long hair usually have a confident, unique, and rebellious mindset," I said.

"I don't know many men with long hair. I'm a barber," his smile broadened.

"Yes, but apart from Samson the Hero's hair, is there any other energetic, spiritual meaning to hair in the Bible?"

"Sure," Benny stopped the motion of his scissors for a moment and focused. Tom smiled at me from the mirror.

"First of all, according to the Kabbalah, hair is made of very limited light, so it doesn't hurt when it's cut."

"In that case, do most people have limited, black-tinted hair?" I smiled.

Benny continued gravely, "in the Bible, beards and side curls have spiritual significance and so it is forbidden to cut them."

"Forbidden to shave them with a knife," I said confidently.

"And for good reason because, according to the Kabbalah, the enlightenment of wisdom is found in the beard."

I remembered hearing about this once before and I nodded. I was slightly disappointed that he was stating what I already knew.

"Did you know that impurity sticks to hair, and so Priests were once commanded to shave their entire body before a purification ceremony, including their eyebrows?"

"So women and men from all over the world who remove all their body hair are, in fact, constantly preparing for a purification ceremony without removing their eyebrows..." I was amused, but Benny remained grave.

"You're probably wondering why, if one has to remove all the hair, God gave us hair to begin with?" He insisted.

"Why indeed?" I was curious.

"In order to attain grace and closeness with God, preparation is necessary together with labor and a meaningful process of refinement and purification bring Man to his highest virtue."[17]

---

17. From the words of Avraham Yitzchak HaCohen Kook.

"Hair removal is a meaningful process of refinement?" I hadn't thought of it that way.

"We perform physical acts that may appear ordinary, but their effect is spiritual."

"I totally agree with you," I marveled.

A young man came into the barber shop talking on his smartphone.

He nodded to Benny.

"How are you?" Benny welcomed him, "I'll be with you in a minute."

Tom's hair was soon perfectly cut. He looked older. It was a peep at the man to come.

"That looks so nice," I enthused.

Benny took Tom down from the chair. "Who wants a surprise?" He asked, clapping his hands.

"Me," cried Ethan. He was expecting it.

Benny took two packets of plastic Mikado pick-up-sticks and gave them to the boys. I took out my credit card and put it on the counter.

"Itchy," Tom scowled with discomfort and he scratched his neck. He was experiencing the tickly sense of short hair for the first time.

"We're going home to shower," I soothed him, formally adding: "the hair cutting ceremony is over and we're now moving on to purification through water in a bath full of toys."

*Additional Aspects of
Energy Hair Experiments*

Natural Straightening

"Are you still talking to your hair?" I asked Lia while removing the plates from the table after lunch.

"Mom, don't pressure me because of your book," she replied.

"You're the one who wanted straight hair like your friends," I said, putting a pile of dishes into the sink.

"How come I'm the only one in the family with curly hair?"

I stood in front of her. "Do you know what makes your hair curly?"

"No, I don't know. Nobody in the family has frizzy hair."

"I went online and read that curly hair grows out of a flat follicle at a curved angle from the scalp. Curly hair has tighter Sulphur bonds that make hair curly."

She looked sad. "So there's nothing I can do. For me, every day is a bad hair day. I have to live with this hair for the rest of my life."

"No, you don't have to. If you change your approach towards your hair you can make the pharmacy in your body change the chemistry of your hair. Emotions carry chemical messages in the body that change the chemical composition of the cells. You can cause the Sulphur bonds to loosen. You yourself can straighten your hair."

Lia pursed her lips.

"The physical body is like clay that we mold according to our needs. It is not concrete into which we pour our consciousness."[18]

"What?"

"Russian scientists have done research proving that it is possible to change DNA through the use of words."

"It's hard for me to do that."

"I can help you. I'll talk to your hair. Sit down for a moment; I'll loosen your hair."

Reluctantly, she sat down.

I removed the thin elastic band from her tight ponytail and discovered another, and another..."How many do you use?"

I don't want my hair to move," she grumbled.

"Another one? Four elastic bands? You're overdoing it. I feel as if I'm neutralizing a bomb," I shuddered.

"Mom, stop, you don't understand."

I twisted the last black elastic band to loosen it and her hair burst out in all directions. I ran my fingers through her hair to air it, but it just moved through my fingers and returned to its place. Lia's head looked like a round bush.

"Your hair isn't pleasant to touch. I'll cut it for you," I offered.

She couldn't bear the situation. "No, Mom, that's enough."

"Just a little," I emphasized, going to fetch the scissors.

"Just a little," she demanded, "because otherwise I won't be able to put it up in a ponytail."

---

18. From: "The Nature of Physical Reality, A Seth Book," chapter 10.

"Don't exaggerate, your hair is long." I brought over the large, sharp scissors I use to cut fabric. I cut off about seven centimeters of her hair with enjoyment. A bunch of prickly hair was left in my hand. It seemed like a pom-pom.

"We can make a keyring from it; it's fashionable now."

"Mom!"

"I was joking," I said, hurriedly, binning the bunch of hair.

"Okay, let's begin," I stood behind her. "We need a comb," I told her.

Lia knew she couldn't avoid my decision to treat her hair and went off to her room to fetch a brush.

I brushed her hair with the large brush, encountering stiff resistance from knots.

Lia occasionally let out a shriek of pain. When her hair had no more knots, I caressed it, saying it was "already straight." I stretched her hair and saw it had potential. I imagined it falling straight, soft, and pleasant. I repeated the mantra again and again. I asked Lia to participate in the guided visualization so that she'd be part of the process.

Lia, who was submissive and ready for the possibility of magic, spirituality and science, also prepared herself for reality: "and if it doesn't work, I want a hair straightener. I need something professional for my hair," she made sure to demand.

"You won't need it. I will make your hair fall smoothly."

After I finished treating all her hair, declaring it to be straight, Lia gathered it up. Adele appeared on her way to the kitchen.

"By humanizing all the cells, you'd experience your body as a special community. Your hair follicles will do anything for you. Your hair is waiting for us to talk to it. It thinks about you and feels like you've been let down with its default instruction to grow curly and frizzy."

"May it stop disappointing me and grow straight."

"If you'd rise above the feeling of a solid body requiring nourishment, cleanliness and something tasty to snack on, you'd love and appreciate it. You'd feel compassion, love and huge respect for your body which consists of trillions of minute, wise units doing sacred work for you twenty-four hours a day."

"Okay Mom, I want to make chocolate chip cookies. Is there any dark chocolate?"

"Did you know that chocolate chip cookies were invented by mistake because the owner of a small American inn added chopped-up bits from a semi-sweet chocolate bar," commented Adele from the kitchen.

"I told you, the American chocolate chips recipe is the tastiest," Lia told me.

"Okay, as long as you make the cookies. The industry uses human hair to reinforce the flavor of cookies and baked goods," I said.

"Yuck," cried Adele.

"I don't care, I need something tasty now," said Lia, taking eggs out of the fridge.

"When I was a little girl, I'd suck on the ends of my hair," I said.

Adele made a face.

"Lia, clean up after yourself," I instructed.

"I'm making cookies for everyone. You clean up."

This arrangement suited us both.

Hair Garden

I went out onto the balcony and sat down beside Gabriel.

"What is he talking about?"

"It's a speech from the ceremony for the American Embassy move from Tel Aviv to Jerusalem."

I also watched Gabriel's smartphone. He was excited, "We're living in historic times."

We listened to the President's speech: *"I have determined that it is time to officially recognize Jerusalem as the capital of Israel."* Trump's serious face expressed determination.

A blue tie complemented his suit.

"Do you think that's his own hair?" I wondered out loud.

"Is that what interests you?"

"Yes."

"I believe it's his hair. Look, physically, he's a very strong man."

"He's a very optimistic man."

"What's the connection?"

"I know he read a book on positive thinking when he was young and that it really affected him."

"And -?" Gabriel was mystified.

"Positive energy is directly related to hair."

"He eats meat. That's the connection to his having hair at his age."

"You don't understand," I said.

"What?"

He won't like it.

"One can energetically stop hair from growing and, theoretically, one can also grow hair."

"People suffer more from baldness."

"No, not really. As a woman, I understand the suffering involved in removing hair and so I identify with that suffering. On the other hand, you can identify with baldness in a man. It seems more important to you."

"There are solutions to removing hair, even if they're unpleasant. There is no real solution for hair that disappears from the head," said Gabriel, his eyes still on the screen.

"It's logical, but there is a solution."

Gabriel turned off his smartphone and glanced at the watch on his wrist. He leaned his arms on the railing and waited.

"Do you know how hair is structured?"

"Like tiles, one on top of another."

How did he know?

"I've thought about it. Baldness probably feels like living in a home without a roof; like being homeless inside your house. It has a bad effect on many balding people, making them feel unconfident and even depressed. Balding or thinning hair isn't a voluntary choice for men and women," I added.

"Obviously, and you have a cure for cancer."

"Yes, to me it is obvious and theoretically simple."

"You merely have a theory and a romantic attitude to life."

"My theory is just as perfect as removing hair energetically. It probably works, but nobody seems to have tried it."

"Apart from you, with an imagined theory."

"But it is easy to understand that anyone interested in seeing the magnificence of all his hair again must develop an awareness and understanding of the grace, generosity, and Divine abundance inherent in the nature of the body."

Gabriel clasped his hands.

"I can explain it to you briefly and technically."

Gabriel gazed at me.

"The body prints 3D hair and baldness is caused by a change in programming," I said lightly.

"Are you serious?" He shook his head. "The cause of baldness is mainly genetic," he stated confidently.

"That's true, but you know what that means? Stress activates a genetic hormone that causes baldness. There is also a type of baldness that is caused by an autoimmune disease. Most people think that the roots of their hair die, but what actually happens is that the growth time of hair shortens and, later on, growth slows down to such an extent that what we see is baldness. But the good news is that genetics and illness can be positively changed."

"Yeah, sure."

"The visual process of balding is similar to the process I went through of energetically removing hair. The hair becomes thin, light, and weak and then it gets shorter. Small areas of baldness form until all the hair stops growing. So why not try the reverse process? It's preferable to all the methods offered today."

"Hair implants sound horrifying to me," said Gabriel.

"Some people get a hair tattoo, which is no solution; it's a drawing. There's an electrical device that stimulates some follicles and a pill with the side effect of a decreased libido."

Gabriel looked piercingly at me. "Do you want to see a movie?"

"Science fiction?"

"Yes," he replied.

"Have you noticed that recently all science fiction movies we've seen are about journeys to distant stars in the galaxy and the possibility of our colonizing those stars because in the future we won't be able to live on earth?"

"It's known as the apocalypse."

"It's extraordinary what cinema culture puts into people's minds. I tell you, when people are tired of looking for remote solutions, they'll have no alternative but to dig down deep within themselves."

Gabriel did not respond; I'd lost contact with him. I closed the subject: "just let me say one thing: whoever experiments has a different comprehension of the body and life."

A Head of Grass

On the right side of the broad road near the Ra'anana City Junction to the north is a large sign with a huge image of a cannabis leaf and the inscription:

"You won't find *this* here, but you will find everything else."

I thought of it as a brave and amusing advertisement. It made me want to find out more about the place and, maybe, buy a plant on the way.

When I got home, I walked upstairs and reached the front door with difficulty. I was holding a box which contained a large bag of soil, fertilizer, two hanging baskets, mint and stevia seedlings, and two bald, grass heads.

Putting on disposable gloves, I arranged soil mixed with good fertilizer in the baskets on the kitchen table. I planted the mint and stevia seedlings and hung the baskets from the large railing at the closed balcony window in the living room.

The boys burst in noisily with Gabriel following.

"Hel-lo," I called to them.

"What's that?" Ethan immediately noticed the grass heads.

Gabriel put the boys' kindergarten bags on the floor and noticed the gardening packet.

"That's nice; what have you brought?" he asked.

"Mint seedlings for your tea," I pointed at the hanging baskets.

"Great," he didn't bother to examine them. "I'm off to work. Say goodbye," he addressed the little ones, but they were standing in front of the bald grass heads. Gabriel exchanged a glance with me, nodded, and left. I gave the boys a short lesson on agriculture and spirituality.

"That's a grass head. When you water it, grass grows out of its head."

"Cool," said Ethan.

"Cool," repeated Tom and touched the grass head.

"I've brought you little green watering cans."

"I want a green watering can," Ethan enthused.

I filled it with water at the sink and let them water the head.

"When will it grow?" asked Ethan.

"It takes at least a few days. But if you want to hasten the process and make the grass grow tall and strong, you can tell the grass to grow."

"Like you talked to Lia's hair?" asked Ethan.

"Yes, grass, grow tall," I said with intention to the seedlings inside the bald heads.

Ethan cooperated. "Grass, grow tall," he said, gazing at the unmoving head.

"Grass, grow tall," I continued the energetic irrigation.

"Grass, grow tall," said Ethan.

"Grass, grow tall," chimed Tom.

Balance

With the passing of time and Gabriel's repeated comments, I gradually internalized the notion that an orderly house directly affects how one feels and that external energy affects the internal state of one's mind. It was important to me to change my attitude. It filtered into me and I had to make more effort. I bought brown woven baskets and solid plastic containers as well as several other pretty round storage containers in varying sizes.

"Adele, Lia," I called, loaded with large bags.

"We're in our room," Adele replied.

The girls were in the same position they were in during the morning when I left with the boys.

"We're starting to tidy up."

"What?" called Lia.

"Put down the phone," I demanded.

"I'm not watching movies, I'm reading Wattpad."

"Which is?"

"An application for writing and reading stories," replied Lia.

"Okay, we're now tidying Marie Kondo style," I said, putting the bags down on the floor.

"Why did I tell you about that show?" Lia protested at

having her right to do nothing taken away from her during the summer vacation.

"It's an excellent show; exactly for messy people like us. Although we aren't hoarders, we don't have a method for keeping things tidy in the house. Besides, I like the way Marie tells people to talk to their clothes and thank them before getting rid of them. It's nice to see people working with this method. It makes the notion of talking to hair appear much more normal."

Adele switched from a lying position to sitting up. "Some people talk to their cars to get the engine running. Does it make the car start? No!"

I didn't want to start a discussion. "Come on, we're doing origami with your clothes. All your clothes out of the closet and on the bed, now."

Reluctantly, they cooperated. Adele's pile of clothes was relatively larger than Lia's. She did the work alone, occasionally asking me for advice regarding a garment that was too small for her and was hard to give away. Lia primarily watched from the side as I did the work for her. An hour later, accompanied by interruptions from the little ones, the closets appeared as tidy as a catalog of closets in a store.

"That is so nice," I marveled, gazing at the boxes lying one beside the other, filled with carefully folded clothes. The sight calmed the body and soul.

"If you respect your clothes and belongings, you'll respect yourselves," I told them lightly. I was satisfied, but they at once fell back on their beds with their smartphones.

"Wait, Lia," I said.

"But, we're done," she protested.

I left the room, returning with a large white bag. I put it on her bed.

She peeped inside. "You've bought me a professional hair straightener," she said excitedly.

"Yes, you decided that you didn't want to continue the treatment. I can't keep persuading you. It doesn't work by force. It's a pity that you don't understand that the hair treatment we did is a gradual process. The stages prepare you for a high state of reality and joy that you can internalize as a part of your existence. It's a shame you lost patience; there have been substantial results."

"Mom, I'll manage just fine with the hair straightener, thank you." She hugged me.

"You could have been the first in history to straighten your hair energetically."

"I can live with that," she said indifferently, "but if you want to know, I've been inspired by you and am writing stories on Wattpad. I already have five likes." she smiled broadly.

"Great. what are you writing about?"

"I'm writing science fiction for kids," she said happily.

"Excellent," I said, looking at her hair that was tied back.

"Mom, I'm not writing a science fantasy about hair."

I sighed. "Okay. In any case, people will probably think that's what *I* am doing."

The End of the Experiment

I examined my face in the mirror. Seven days had passed since I'd removed the last short hairs from my upper lip. Now, it was smooth, hairless, bright, and clean.

I was excited from having reached the finish line, but the joy filling me was mixed with the sadness of parting from the treatment, which really had succeeded in getting rid of the hair. My face was radiant and I waited for Gabriel to return that evening.

"I've finished the treatment. I can now formally say that my theory is proven," I declared as he stood on the threshold. Gabriel gazed round at the tidy home as if he were having a hard time believing he was in the right house.

The kitchen table was clean and the toys were organized and categorized in boxes in a beehive cabinet.

"You never had a mustache," said Gabriel.

"Only you could say something like that."

"I never noticed that you had a mustache," he insisted.

There was no point in arguing.

"The experiment worked perfectly. My theory has

been proven. Hair does indeed respond to energetic talking and gradually disappears from one treatment to another."

"How long did it take?"

"Two years."

"Isn't that a long time?"

"It's a really long time, but it's complicated. There are other areas of the body where I got faster results. I felt a difference in the feelings operating within me."

Gabriel, who had already entered the house, gave me a disappointed look. "How many treatments were there in numbers? People are impatient, you know. People always do less than what is necessary and if they don't have to do a thing, that's what they'll prefer to do."

"The table I made got wet from the boys' splashing in the bath, so I don't have a precise number of self-treatments. In any case, treatments always consist of factors like the thickness of hair and the power of the energy transferred to it."

"Give me an average time."

"People can get rid of hair in up to six months; it depends on the frequency of the treatments and the accompanying emotions."

Gabriel looked at me in astonishment. He went into the kitchen and took a raspberry and chia shake out of the freezer.

"Apart from that, removing hair by laser takes more than a year. Some are treated with laser for years, so if we look at it in terms of time measurement, removing hair through energy is a clear winner," I added.

"But you still haven't proven it."

I was angry. "You know what? I don't have to prove

it. Einstein didn't prove his theory about the deflection of starlight; a delegation of British scientists managed to photograph a solar eclipse and they were the ones who proved it. And I am not talking about distant starlight, but something much closer and more concrete that anyone can try. Besides, Einstein's famous equation $E=mc^2$ accurately explains the issue," I said.

Gabriel sucked the shake through the straw and shifted his weight from one foot to the other.

"The equation explains that energy can transform into matter and matter can transform into energy," I added.

"Your thinking is too abstract," said Gabriel.

I dropped into a nearby kitchen chair.

Gabriel sat down opposite me. "Abraham was the first to believe in the abstract. He gazed at the stars and later concluded that God is not matter, but a spiritual force that activates the world. He was the first to tell idol worshipers how ridiculous it was to bow down to statues. His life mission was to teach people that God is the only invisible force that is active in the world."

I wasn't sure what he was getting at.

"Do you think God would prefer people to remove hair energetically?"

"Obviously I do," I burst out passionately. Pulling myself together, I continued quietly, "God told Moses to speak to the rock so that water would come out of it. God wanted everyone to see how unique He was and Moses, instead of speaking, struck the rock twice. God was disappointed that Moses didn't believe in Him. I assume that God would prefer us to talk to our hair instead of behaving violently. God gave us simple tools and we have them in our hands all the time, available in sound waves and a heartbeat."

"If so, you could be the CEO of Energy Hair Removal." Gabriel came up with a job for me.

I didn't understand how I became the CEO of something.

"You can sell it if you believe in it," he explained.

"I'm not selling a theory. It isn't a gimmick. It's about important, sensitive, and revolutionary knowledge."

"I don't sell furniture. I only advise people and they buy it because they believe me. They see my professionalism in the field," he said.

"And that is what I will do. I will advise people based on my experience. I hope that many brave and intelligent people will try it, because only the evidence of many people will report positive results will prove my theory to the world." I said.

Gabriel noisily sucked up the last of the shake together with bubbles of air from the bottom of the glass.

"So do what you can and pray," he concluded.

Doubts

The grass heads grew. Green, fresh and tall, they stood on the computer table in the living room. Things develop better when you relate to them. Everyone seems to need attention and admiration of their existence.

Gabriel worked the morning shift that day. The girls were in school and the boys were in kindergarten.

The house was peaceful.

I moved the mouse and pressed "print." The printer came to life; the ink head made dragging, screeching sounds, then stopped. It drew page after page and began to move right and left. The sound of printing echoed in the living room and after a hundred and fifty pages an alarming silence reigned.

In my hand, I held the product of the time I spent with the words I'd uttered and formed.

I'd waited so long for this. I straightened the papers and held them close to me. After some time, I put them in the last drawer of the dresser that matched the wooden computer table. I closed the drawer and went to the kitchen. I returned, opened the drawer, and took out the pages. Was I mad? After all, I hadn't written for the drawer. A drawer has no hair.

I laid the pages at the far corner of the table, away from the children. I felt restless. What shall I do now? Send it to a publisher again? I didn't feel ready. I had cold feet. I was afraid of another rejection.

***

I made an effort to steady my hand. I gently inserted a red Mikado stick under the blue stick and tossed it into the air. The stick flew behind the laptop on the table. Gabriel was sitting in front of it. He glanced at me, bothered by the disturbance. I smiled an apology.

I inserted the red Mikado stick under the yellow one on top of a pile of several other sticks, but this time my hand trembled and I moved a few sticks. I was tired of playing.

"I don't know what to do," I said.

Gabriel was absorbed in a 3-D sketch of a closet.

"I don't know what to do."

"About what?" He moved the cordless laptop mouse.

"About the book," I answered.

"What about it?" He strained his eyes in an effort to focus on the sketch.

"Oh, I don't know. I've finished writing it."

"About time," he responded.

I daydreamed. "There are a lot of books in bookstores."

"What did you expect to find there?" He looked at me.

I bit my lip. "I've decided not to send the book to a publisher. If anything, I'll publish it myself."

"I'm wondering", he said, leaning back in his chair and giving me a penetrating look, "if you have Graphomania?"

"What's that?" I was uneasy about his answer.

"Great enthusiasm for literary writing without any talent for it."

"Thank you," I was insulted.

"In any case, if you publish it yourself, it will cost a lot of money," said Gabriel.

I was silent and pricked my hand with a Mikado stick.

"I won't take a bet on the book," he stated, again focusing on the laptop screen.

I felt my throat tighten. "You mean you won't take a bet on me?"

I sounded a little hoarse.

He looked up at me again. "How can I? You never completely finish anything. You've neglected your painting. You've done all sorts of courses and nothing came from any of them."

"But it's different now. This is different. It's me, don't you understand?"

"No," he said, and went back to the screen.

"You could have been more supportive. I'm afraid of reactions from people with strong opinions, and I don't like feeling exposed. I enjoy being as anonymous as I can be. I could happily live seeing while being invisible. Publishing a book with an innovative concept is no simple matter, I don't know what to do."

"So don't do anything," declared Gabriel.

I couldn't meet his eyes.

"Alright, I won't!" I raised my voice.

Gabriel looked up. "So don't."

"I won't," I shouted. The words echoed inside me and without thinking, I swept all the Mikado sticks off the table and hurried away to the bedroom.

What Does One Do with a Theory

I sat down on a small, square, wooden chair like the ones in the children's kindergarten in front of the boys' bed, and hugged a book to myself. That afternoon I went into a bookstore in the local mall, looking for a new book for the children. The book stood out because of its size, white cover, and pleasant illustration of a boy with an egg. I looked through it. The illustrations were attractive and the text was brief, light, and readable. I thought the boys would love it and I had a feeling that I'd also like the book.

The boys were fooling around in the store and I hurriedly bought it. I decided to read it with them.

"I've bought you a new book," I said, "come on, into bed," I told them.

"Show me," asked Ethan, coming over to me. He looked intently at the illustration on the cover: a boy smiling at a golden egg with a crown on his head.

"Is that the *Egg that Disguised Itself?*"[19] he asked.

"No," I replied.

---
19. *The Egg that Disguised Itself* written and illustrated by Dan Pagis, Am Oved Publishers

"Is it a surprise egg?" he tried again.

I smiled. "No, it's an egg that symbolizes an idea. But you are right, a new idea can be a surprise of sorts."

The Big Bang melody was playing in the pocket of my tailored black coat. A call came from "Gabriel, a smiley with hearts in its eyes."

"Hi, I'm just reading a story to the children," I said at once.

"Great, I'll be home earlier today. Shall we go out?"

"Yes", I was surprised. "Bye for now," I hurried to end the conversation. My mind was on the children and the new book.

The boys got onto the bed and I read the name of the book:

"*What Do You Do With an Idea? by* Kobi Yamada.*"*[20]

I opened the book in front of them so they could easily see the illustrations of the characters.

I read the story about the boy and the egg. Amazed, Ethan and Tom followed the concept of the developing egg that grew larger and larger in the time between one page and another. At this point, I realized I was reading my own story of recent years to myself. The story was about me. I was that child, and the egg symbolized my theory. The story detailed precisely all the stages I went through from the moment the idea took root in my mind. It reminded me of the road I took from the moment of my fear of what others would say, to the moment the theory became an important and inseparable part of my life. I identified with the brave and loving connection forged between the child

---

20. *What Do You Do With an Idea?* by Kobi Yamada, translated by Yehuda Atlas, Celanter Books, 2015

and the concept of the egg and was moved when the idea manifested and connected with everything in the world.

At the end of the story, the boy understands: *an idea can change the world.*

My heart beat fast.

I also understood: my theory could change the world.

I will never know how far my theory will go, whom it will touch, or how it will affect them. I hope, it will beneficially affect some man or woman. It is both my duty and my right to convey what is inside of me. I remembered I had a task to complete.

Ethan sat up in bed. "Now read us *We Are in a Book*."[21]

He brought me swiftly back to earth.

I was too excited. "It's late. Enough for today, bedtime."

"Then read us *The Giving Tree*."[22] He begged so sweetly.

"Okay," I relented, unable to refuse.

After the story, the boys were mellow and ready to go to sleep. I kissed them and once they were asleep, I went into the kitchen.

Adele emerged from her room. "Great, you read them stories."

I hushed her. "Enough. I've learned my lesson, don't start."

---

21. *We are in a Book* by Mo Willems, translated by Meira Fitan, Tel-May publishing house, 2016.
22. *The Giving Tree* by Shel Silverstein, translated: Yehuda Meltzer, "Adam" publishing house, 1980.

"The stories you read to me and Lia were the shortest in the world: 'once upon a time, nothing happened,' or 'once there was a princess who didn't need a prince, the end,'" Adele insisted on reminding me of my shame.

"I was a young, single parent and didn't understand the importance of reading stories to children. I've frequently apologized for not reading you more ordinary bedtime stories, so what do you want?"

"An apology always improves how I feel," she replied.

"I didn't really make you think one doesn't need a prince, right?"

"Right; we knew it was a joke."

"I'm really sorry," I apologized with all my heart.

Adele's face expressed satisfaction.

"I'm thinking of having short bangs, what do you say?" she asked, spreading the ends of her hair on her forehead in an attempt to see what it would look like.

I looked at her. "It will suit you," I responded.

"Did you know that the Russian word 'Chupchik' means a small strand of hair on the front of the head?"

"Really? I always thought 'chupchik' was the spout of an old-fashioned kettle which they used to boil water over the gas. When I was a little girl, we had a metal one at home."

Adele pushed back the ends of her hair. "It sounds like an antique."

"Yes, but I loved that kettle. I liked listening to its whistle."

"Look at me," she asked and stood, her head erect. I looked at her long boots that were the same style as mine, suede with wool at the top. While mine were brown, hers were black.

"You're taller. It's working for you, bravo!" I said, proud of her experimentation with her own energy treatment.

"I met a friend from school. She didn't understand how I'd grown so quickly, while she stayed short." She smiled to herself and changed the subject: "I took all sorts of photographs. Tell me which ones are nice."

Adele took out her smartphone.

"Nice," I responded to the picture I saw.

"Unnatural," I said at the sight of duck lips.

"That profile picture looks artificial," I gave my opinion.

"Isn't it pretty?" Adele was hurt.

"You want me to tell you the truth, don't you?"

"Then what shall I upload to Instagram?"

"The one where you're smiling," I replied as I chose for her.

"It's a terrible picture and it's blurred."

"It's a wonderful photograph; you're smiling naturally."

The door opened and Gabriel came in.

"Hi," I said.

"Are you coming?" he asked.

"Where?"

"Come on, let's go."

"We're going out," I told Adele and instructed her, "keep an eye on the boys."

"Enjoy," she said as she went into her room while examining the photographs.

I was wearing a maroon sweater and a short, soft, blue skirt. I felt tall and full of energy.

***

We got into the car and slammed the doors. Gabriel made a sharp U-turn.

"Tell me, how long has it been since you started writing?" He asked while watching the road ahead.

"Two years. It feels like a lifetime."

"You stuck to it."

"And all that time I focused on a theory that shatters the premise that body hair should be treated as mere matter. And to think that medicine once separated body and mind..."

"René Descartes."

"Today, most people know that there is a strong connection between the body and mind and that they are mutually beneficial," I said.

"I am totally in agreement," said Gabriel.

I was silent in the face of his approval.

"I think you should go all the way with the book," he said.

"You think so?"

Gabriel took my hand and said, "I'm certain!"

I didn't know what to say. I looked out at the passing store windows.

"So, you've finished writing. Now what?"

"Now I'm supposed to find an editor."

He nodded.

"I spoke to Hannah not long ago and she told me that women have commented that her eyebrows always look clean. It's hard not to notice because she has a relatively large space between her eyebrows."

Gabriel was silent. He apparently didn't know what to do with the information.

"She used to go to a beautician to remove facial hair, but in recent months she's been standing in front of the mirror in the living room, plucking her eyebrows and telling the hair to stop growing. She didn't care if any family members were around." I was amused.

"So others have succeeded too?"

"Of course, but she told me that her daughter Ruth didn't succeed. Ruth told her hair to stop growing, and immediately afterwards she told it to grow, funny child."

"How did you explain it to her?"

"When I was visiting, I explained a little bit about the theory and less about the feeling during treatment."

He seemed focused. "Maybe you should write a book on hair removal for children."

I looked at him in disbelief and tried to think. "In the end, all physical theories must be simple so that any child can understand,"[23] I said.

We were silent.

"How come you're supporting me on this?"

"Listen, it's interesting. On Saturday, when you took the boys to the park, I read the book, *The Secret Life of Plants*. What happens in the book is amazing," he said.

---

23. Einstein.

"Have you noticed that the plant is getting smarter now? It's growing along the narrow wall under the railing so that we won't see it spread. That plant is really cunning but it creates a decoration – a beautiful external frame for the balcony."

Gabriel turned right at the lights on Hagibborim Street. We were traveling south and I guessed we were on our way to the Feinberg House, the first private home in Hadera, which became a museum and a restaurant. Gabriel turned left at the square and stopped in front of a white entrance gate.

"I don't feel like sitting in a restaurant," I said quietly.

Gabriel drove on and the destination didn't matter to me. He turned around and left the city, traveling north until we reached the sea front at Caesarea.

"Do you remember our first date?" Gabriel gazed at me.

"Yes; it was in the car, at the sea in Herzliya. But at the time, you had red wine and disposable glasses."

"We could have gone into the restaurant." He silenced the engine, released his seat belt, and relaxed in his seat.

We remained sitting in the car. The darkness was soft. We talked, looking out at the stormy mid-winter white foam. At a certain point, my body hurt from sitting without moving and I became restless. Turning around, I rested my knees against the seat and my back against the glove compartment.

"If you had the opportunity to do anything in the world, what would you do?"

Gabriel had often asked me this question.

"I'd read a good book," I answered, examining his response. He grimaced with dissatisfaction.

"Nothing else comes to mind," I apologized.

"In that case, publishing your book should be your best experience," said Gabriel.

I turned my head away and looked straight ahead at the darkness spreading beyond the back window.

"What is frightening you?" he asked.

"What if I'm merely a tiny particle in the world that no one will think of measuring."

"Any book you write will be interesting."

"You yourself refused to read the guide."

"When the book is ready and has a cover, I will read it. Promise."

I shook my head. "But everything could suddenly change."

"It's about time, don't you think?" He yawned.

"I hope everything turns out okay."

"The most important thing is never, ever give up." He said decisively, continuing, "Soon, the whole world will know that one can talk to body hair" He tried to extract an explicit promise from me.

"Not the whole world - just a part of it," I said cautiously.

"But it is still a real part, with real people," he said.

A shudder of excitement and fear gripped me. "Are you trying to pressure me?" I felt a chill on my arms. I exposed my left arm. "My hair is standing on end," I said.

"Your hair is saluting you," said Gabriel leaning towards me. "It encourages you..." He whispered.

I burst out laughing.

Gabriel smiled with satisfaction, sat up in his seat, and turned the key in the ignition. He drove backwards in a swift, dizzying turn. The tires rubbed hard against the gravel. I felt relaxed and safe. I remained sitting in the car, facing the opposite direction of the traffic.

The End

How to Remove Hair Through Energy

A Guide

The guide is a source of extra information, and serves as an extension to the book "Razor Free."

The energetic removal of hair constitutes far more than the creation of smooth skin.
- It is intelligent hair removal in the era of spiritual science.
- It is hair removal through the discovery of inner strength.
- It is hair removal that is priceless: Recognition of a collaborative body.

The guide before you includes an explanation of the body's energy, the emotional technique for arresting the hair growth, the stages in the process, and tips for the journey.

This is the quickest, simplest, most qualitative and healthiest way to achieve permanent hair removal.

Being a new and unique niche, it is not mentioned anywhere else.

The guide is meant for women, men, and teens.
1. It is intended for those frequently suffering from the pain and frustration involved in removing hair.
2. The method reduces the pain of plucking to zero.
3. It is intended for any pigment, thickness, or color of hair.
4. It can occur anywhere on the body.
5. It occurs in privacy.
6. It can occur during every season of the year.
7. It is suited for any medical condition. (It is not advisable during pregnancy)
8. It does not require any materials.
9. It is free of charge.

*"If you want to find the secrets
of the universe, think in terms of
energy, frequency, and vibration."*
Nikola Tesla

CONTENTS

Energy, Frequency, and Vibration	185
The Stages of an Emotional Technique	189
Additional Information	195
Stages of Growth Arrest	195
Visualization Isn't Easy	195
Background Noise	196
Large Areas of Hair	196
Minimum Treatment Duration	196
Results According to the Number of Treatments	197
The Condition of the Hair During Treatment	198
Laser	198
Do We have to Talk to Hair?	199
Talking to All Body Hair Simultaneously	199
Tone of Speech	200
In the Beginning	200
Right and Left	200

The Technical Removal of Hair in-between Treatments	201
Side Effects	201
Setting a Time for Treatment	201
Breaks In-Between Treatments	201
Frequency of Treatments	202
Treatment Follow-up	202
Permanent Treatment	202
Sweet Hairy Children	203
The next generation: Epigenetics	203
DIT – Do It Together	205
Questionnaire	207
Tips	211
Emotion at Work	213

Energy, Frequency, and Vibration

The body consists of about fifty trillion cells.

Existing within the deep internal layer of the cells is a world of energy, vibration, and frequency.

The energy constitutes power, vibrating movement, and a frequency that constitutes rhythm.

Each cell in the body has a specific vibration frequency through which it expresses its energetic essence, color, texture, and function, etc.

Our body consists of energy patterns that shape the various parts of the body.

If there is a change in an energy pattern, there will be a change in physical biology. In order to generate a significant change in a hair cell, we need to act on the vibrational level of the cell. When we change the vibration of hair growth, the hair will stop growing.

It's that simple.

How do we change vibration? We direct emotion.

Every thought, emotion, and word has a vibration and a representative energetic frequency.

The Body-Mind connection is on the continuum between the vibration and chemical response of the cell. Emotion is an energetic message. It is a prescription of sorts borne by chemical compounds secreted into the bloodstream, which arrive at their destination like messengers, feeding the cells with information and action.

The higher the intensity of the emotion, the higher the dose of chemical substance released and the greater its physical effect.

For example: the emotion of fear releases adrenaline; the emotion of love releases dopamine.

What emotion will formulate the precise chemical substance that will arrest the growth of hair?

Frequency constitutes the body's mother tongue.

We translate frequencies into emotions. We do it automatically without being aware of it. The emotional system gives us the precise diagnosis at each moment with regard to where we stand on the frequency scale: high on the positive scale or low on the negative scale.

A positive emotion indicates that we are going in the right direction for manifesting something good. A negative emotion indicates that we are moving in the direction of manifesting something that isn't good.

Consequently, we will always strive for a positive emotion generally on a high frequency and particularly during an energetic hair removal treatment.

Notice the words predominating in your thoughts with regard to hair removal:

"I'm sick of removing hair," "disgusting hair," "why do I have such bad genes."

Stop holding such negative thought patterns. Turn your thoughts into positive ones: "hair is a natural part of the body," I honor the presence of hair," hair will stop growing for me."

Think of the words "smooth skin." Positive words produce a positive emotion inside of us. Think about the body part you most want to be permanently hairless. Imagine that part smooth and hairless forever. This will generate heightened emotion in you.

The best way to achieve heightened emotion is through a mental image. After all, we know that one image is worth a thousand words.

The highest frequencies are joy and gratitude. When we turn to these frequencies and feel them within our body, we achieve the best and speediest results.

When we experience pleasure and joy – when our hair has **already** stopped growing - the frequency of the regular hair-growth pattern is disrupted. The hair pattern loses its balance, breaks down, and stops growing.

Removal of hair by laser takes at least ten treatments over approximately a year and a half.

The laser cannot bypass the biological clock, or in other words the cyclical nature of hair, because it treats the material – the hair itself – by burning it down to the follicle. Laser treatment is limited by the nature of the hair. It has other limitations as well.

In contrast, energetic treatment is free from the limiting effects of biological time on hair. According to quantum physics, the possibility that hair will energetically stop growing exists solely in the present. We don't have to arrest hair growth, but rather we can choose a growth-arrest mode.

Thus, when the shift is profoundly energetic at a vibrational level, hair is instantly able to go into pause mode and, at the 'press of an emotional button,' it will rapidly cease growing.

The joy of choosing a positive result is the ultimate, internal "laser" for permanently removing hair.

The Stages of an Emotional Technique

Stage 1 – Breathing
Stage 2 – Imagination
Stage 3 – Speaking Energetically

Inhale slowly through the nose and slowly exhale through the mouth.

Breathing relieves tension, making us stop, focus, and be present in the moment.

Imagine the body part permanently smooth and hairless.

Emotionally ignore the current reality of the hair. Instead, focus on your desired solution.

The imagination reduces the intellectual gap between reality and vision and helps us strongly feel the final result which leads to the arrest of hair growth.

The imagination plays a large, essential, and significant part in the process of removing intellectual resistance.

Imagination constitutes a higher concentration of energy, flow, and conductive frequency of electromagnetic electricity in the body, which guarantees faster results.

This occurs in contrast to emotional resistance that causes internal tension, the slowing down of the electric conductive frequency, and fulfillment.

Imagination accelerates the final result because in our vision, we are already an intrinsic part of it.

Poor imagination – observe and touch the skin of the body part, and enjoy and appreciate the pleasant, smooth sensation. Think what fun it is that the skin is **already** smooth and hairless.

Allow yourself to experience excitement and a sense of peace flowing through your blood as well as a pleasant feeling that your hair has permanently stopped growing.

Sense a cleansing and perfect beauty. Feel comfort, warmth, and joy.

Be grateful.

Rich imagination – use physical images from your inner emotional world.

An effect like the wonder at a surrealistic science fiction video will be engraved, burned and enacted within us, making a strong impression with frequencies of joy, wonder, excitement, and enthusiasm.

The richer our imagination, the faster the result will be.

Examples of Guided Visualization

Imagine a powerful and sophisticated device that makes hair stop growing in an instant. Turn it on and pass it over the surface of the body part. Instantly, you will see that the hair becomes increasingly finer and the energy of the hair is completely weakened; its structure blurs and breaks down as it vanishes into the depths of the cells which become energetically void of hair follicles. You envision the skin of the body part like a field of empty hair cells. The peace and quiet of a cell factory has peacefully stopped producing hair, leaving behind a body part with a layer of smooth and perfect skin.

You are filled with satisfaction, joy, comfort, and gratitude.

Remain for as long as possible in the moments of joy and ecstasy at the creation of eternal beauty.

Repeat what you have imagined for as many times as you can and for a as long as this gives you pleasure.

***

Imagine an advanced, transparent bio-tech switch sticker. You stick it on the body part. Press the switch, and all hair instantly vanishes. You are happy and wonder how easily your skin becomes smooth. Press the switch again; the hair reappears. Play several times by switching the hair on and off.

Feel how simple it is to control hair.

When you are ready, press once more and switch off the hair energy forever.

The body part remains smooth and hairless. It is clean, beautiful, and perfect.

Remove the switch sticker, crumple it up, and throw it in the garbage. Now, after switching off the hair and throwing out the sticker, you are happy: it is impossible for the hair to grow again, and the skin remains permanently smooth. This is the new and permanent state of the body part. You feel relief, comfort, joy and satisfaction.

***

Your indication that the guided visualization works is the accompanying feeling of joy. The more joyful and excited you are, the more effective the energetic action will be.

After the guided visualization, with the mental and emotional image still reverberating within you, you are in an ideal situation to talk to hair.

Talk to your hair with the knowledge generated by the image you created in your imagination. Speak from a sense of affiliation, compassion, and respect.

Speak positively in the present.

Words connect energy and matter.

The words and text with which you choose to express yourself aren't important. It is the intention that matters.

Speak through the emotion created during the guided visualization when you saw the mental image of beauty, pleasure, festivity, and excitement. Acknowledge the new situation: your hair has already permanently stopped growing.

Possible mantras:

"You have stopped growing."

"Hair, stop growing."

"You have stopped growing from within."
"You have stopped."
"You have already stopped."
"I have smooth skin forever."
"My skin is smooth."
"The [body part] is permanently smooth and hairless."

Another possibility:

Increase the energy frequency vibration by choosing layers of words in an ascending order of excitement.

"I allow the hair to stop growing on the [body part],"
"Hair, stop growing."
"Hair, you have stopped growing."
"I know you have stopped growing."
"All the hair has stopped growing."
"How wonderful!"
"I am so happy that you have stopped growing."
"You have completely stopped growing."
"You have now stopped growing."
"You have stopped growing from within."
"I have a beautiful, hairless spot."
"I have smooth skin."
"Smooth skin forever."
"I'm happy about my smooth skin."
"Well done, hair cells."
"I appreciate the stopping of hair growth."
"Thank you."

If at any stage of talking to hair you ask yourself what the hell you're doing, you've probably lost contact with your image. Connect immediately with the last image you created and the joy of feeling like your hair has stopped growing. This will facilitate an easy return to talking to your hair with feeling and the clear knowledge that your hair has indeed stopped growing.

That's it!

You have acted emotionally and guided the vibration of the hair. Biology has changed accordingly. The hair stops growing at once in accordance with the degree of emotion you have created. You will not see immediate results because we don't live in such a fast and energetic nano-reality. All that is left is for you to believe that **the vibration precedes physical proof.** Don't wait for the hair to change form in order to be sure or satisfied; be happy in the present.

Be glad that you have done the treatment and felt what you wished to feel. This is the measure of success.

What ensues is not up to you, but fulfillment is inevitable.

Continue your daily routine with general optimism.

Later on, when you see results and know that you yourself achieved this, there will be great ongoing satisfaction and pleasure in your smooth skin.

Additional Information

Stages of Growth Arrest
- Hair will become fine, weak, and dryer. It will have a slightly curly appearance.
- Naturally long hair will be easy to pull out. The hair will painlessly "jump" into your fingers. You will also be able to pluck hair painlessly from intimate body parts. Pluck hair painlessly from your nostrils.
- Long hairs will grow shorter.
- Bald patches will appear and these areas will expand with frequent treatments.
- For those who shave: hair will grow back softer and less prickly to the touch. The itching that results from shaving will be less irritating until it stops completely.
- The hair may appear longer than usual. There is no need for alarm; this might happen about twice during the process.
- Some hairs may appear white at the tips.

Visualization Isn't Easy
If you have difficulty with visualization, you can talk directly to your hair without a mental image.

Try to feel and experience the words you utter when formulating the desired result.

You can find inspiration in a picture of a woman with smooth skin.

Background Noise
It is possible to talk to hair when there is background noise – no matter if this is heard while removing hair with a designated device, music, or background discussion.

Hair receives the vibration of emotion, and if the noise doesn't distract you the background noise is not a problem. There is no need for complete silence during the treatment; you can have music in the background if you wish.

Large Areas of Hair
Treat places like arms, thighs, calves, back, and belly.

It isn't easy to talk to hair in a large, three-dimensional area, so visualization helps. You can address hair according to the area:

"[Body part], all the hair has stopped growing."

Minimum Treatment Duration
The longer you maintain the visualization, the faster and more significant the effect will be on the hair.

No fixed number of sessions is required for talking to hair.

Make sure that speech is synchronized with emotion. You can stop when you feel satisfied.

However, it is advisable for emotion to operate for at

least a minute or more in order to facilitate the release of sufficient energy momentum for the follicle.

You can use a one-minute hourglass or set the stopwatch on your smartphone so that you know the treatment will take place within a time limit. You will thus be able to free yourself from the pressure of thinking about the number of sessions or the length of time, and you will be able to focus solely on what you are feeling.

If one minute takes emotional effort for you, the minimum amount of time is twenty seconds for each surface of the body part upon which you focus your awareness.

Results According to the Number of Treatments

It isn't only the quantity of treatments that affect hair. The intensity of emotion and intention affect the hair as well. The cleaner, purer, and truer the intention, the lesser the resistance or doubt; the faster you will see results. The measure of the intention is naturally tested by the hair. This measurement is the most accurate. You cannot sue hair for any deviation in measurement that causes a failure to meet the target set by the heart.

If our intention isn't strong enough because we aren't sufficiently "present" until the end result of the vision, it will take longer for hair growth to be arrested.

Remember not to judge your hair or yourselves.

It is always possible to reinforce our intention and come to the energetic hair removal treatment with more preparation, enthusiasm, and motivation by thinking about the desire for reasons that make us feel good about smooth skin and the knowledge that we can affect the energy of our hair.

The speed at which hair growth is arrested depends on our self-confidence and our joy from the results.

The Condition of the Hair During Treatment
You can talk to your hair while plucking or shaving it. Note that if you feel inner resistance, pressure, anger or irritation while removing hair, it would be preferable not to do the energy treatment during the technical removal.

***

You can talk to hair cells without hair being visible. Such times include the use of body cream, showering, or going to bed.

When talking to hair cells, the energy and intention can be deep, internal, and more intense.

***

You can talk to hair even when you aren't removing it at all. You can thus observe the process and, at a certain point, the hair will become dry, causing discomfort. You may feel the need to remove it.

Laser
If you have begun laser treatments and wish to treat your hair energetically, you can stop the laser treatments and switch to energy treatment. It is not advisable to do both treatments simultaneously.

Energy treatment weakens the hair, which negatively affects the results of the laser treatment method.

Do We have to Talk to Hair?
No, but it is preferable. Talking has an additional energetic power that affects the body.

You can meditate, which is known to be an excellent energetic tool which helps you become mindful and bring about change in a state of mental calm and physical relaxation. Meditation reduces mental resistance.

This is not a meditation guide but the general idea is this: Relax the body parts.

Imagine the body part free of hair. Tell your unconscious mind that your hair has stopped growing. Imagine yourselves in your daily lives with smooth skin and feeling good. Be excited and receive your new reality with joy.

Talking to All Body Hair Simultaneously
It would be better to speak to each body part individually particularly at first. Speak to one body part after another rather than the entire body at once. But if you feel comfortable imagining the entire body smooth and you talk to the entire body, do so. The important thing is to feel comfortable, happy, and free-flowing.

Meditation is also suitable for this method, and it is advisable to do it before going to sleep or during any free rest period.

Imagine every body part permanently smooth and hairless.

Dwell comfortably on each body part for some time.

Allow yourself to enjoy a sense of pleasure, confidence, joy, love, freedom, and satisfaction in relation to the fact that your hair has stopped growing.

In your imagination, pass from your feet, calves, thighs, pubis, buttocks and belly to your arms, back, and face.

Tone of Speech

Speak in a normal tone. There is no need to raise your voice to try and "force" the hair to listen. If you have no privacy or if you are embarrassed that someone might hear you, you can whisper. Remember, the important thing is to feel fulfillment.

In the Beginning

It is best to start with a place that has little hair, like the space between the eyebrows or finger joints, the mustache, armpits, or a body part that you are glad and happy to treat. Intense excitement will work quickly in your favor.

Right and Left

We have a natural tendency to act out of habit, like starting a treatment on a particular side of the body, or always talking to hair on the right side before the left. You might see that a particular side responds more quickly. This is because the start of a treatment might be like 'warming up the engine' of energy and intention. If this is the case with you, you could change sides or transmit additional energy to the side you started with.

The Technical Removal of Hair in-between Treatments
At first you can remove hair by any method apart from laser treatments, as mentioned before. If you use the shaving method, pay attention to the change in the hair. After about twenty treatments, try removing hair by plucking, wax, a shaving machine, sugar, or tweezers. Don't worry, in the case of an emergency where you need to shave, it won't hinder the process.

In any case, find something that works well and suits you.

Side Effects
The energetic removal of hair is a perfectly safe process!

There is no need to worry that desired hair, such as hair on your head, eyebrows, or eyelashes will be affected by the treatments and become sparse.

Hair is intelligent. It is aware of the tiniest nuances of thought and feeling.

Hair knows exactly where you intend to stop hair growth.

Energy operates only in the place where you intend for the hair to stop growing. Your focus and vibration is location-specific. Trust the body's intelligence!

Setting a Time for Treatment
Set a specific time for the treatment.

For example, when you're shaving, putting on cream, or going to sleep. Fixing a time in advance for the treatment will obligate you to start and finish the treatment.

Breaks In-Between Treatments
If you take a break between treatments you can always resume the treatment. The hair will wait as an energetic

weakness already formed. The results will be preserved until the next treatment, regardless of the time that has passed since the previous treatment.

Frequency of Treatments
The pace of treatment is personal. It is determined by your need, desire, and ability. The frequency of the treatments depends on you. It could be one to three times a day.

But if you choose to treat yourself several times a day, make sure you aren't trying to hurry the desired results.

Treatment Follow-up
You can mark the number of treatments you do on a graph in order to measure the progress. Consider that the speed of the treatment might differ from one body part to another, especially if the energy of your will and joy differs from one body part to another. Don't check your skin to see if hair has grown. In between treatments, behave as usual and forget about the treatments.

Permanent Treatment
Theoretically, this is a treatment for the permanent arrest of hair growth. Every cell in the body has the qualities of a computer chip.

In his book *The Biology of Belief,* Dr. Bruce Lipton defines the cell of the body as a computer chip. No programming on the chip can be changed unless the chip is reprogrammed. Thus, the vibration programming of the hair cell won't change either, unless it is emotionally redefined.

Sweet Hairy Children

Removing children's body hair usually depends on the parents.

If the children don't wish to remove hair that socially or aesthetically bothers them, it would be better to allow them to grow up and decide for themselves. External beauty is not the main or only goal in life.

If the need to remove hair is initiated by children who are suffering, then a permanent treatment would be preferable in order to avoid dealing with the frequency of need to remove hair at a young age.

A simple explanation of the process for children can be effective and enjoyable. Children like discovering new things about their body. They have a natural, innocent tendency to believe and cooperate, and this could certainly be a special experience for them; one that will foster a more positive self-image and become an empowering "game."

The next generation: Epigenetics
DNA is not fixed or static; it is constantly in a process of change in relation to us, in accordance with every strong emotion that is arrested in our body: fears, trauma, habits and love. These are ingrained in our genes, which is how

we pass on information and genetic influence to the coming generations.

When a man or woman energetically removes hair and achieves a smooth body part or entire body, will this information pass on to their children who will then be born without hair in these places or with less hair?

The emotional process we experience will pass on to whoever inherits our genes; that is, the treatment will have a certain effect. But it is doubtful whether this will find expression in the first generation. In my opinion, it would most likely take several generations and persistence in the energetic removal of hair for our offspring to be born hairless.

Ergo, the energetic removal of hair is a deep-rooted solution that will impact the coming generations.

DIT – Do It Together

The body was born to be free; it doesn't require any external help. A healthy body is supposed to be free of any kind of technological aids. But we human beings are social creatures and we like to do things together.

We can help each other. Reciprocity is good for morale, energy, and motivation. We can choose someone with whom we feel comfortable doing the treatment - someone we trust and whose intentions are good. Someone who is interested in our wellbeing. It can be a friend, a partner.

The person leading the treatment can do a guided visualization regarding the hair, and it is sufficient for the person undergoing treatment to listen actively while emotionally experiencing the process.

It is easier to listen to someone with good intentions and believe in a new and fantastic truth that we are hearing.

It could be a combined spiritual and physiological experience.

You can exchange roles.

It is possible to help each other feel. Two hearts that work together experience quicker results.

Questionnaire

This is a personal indication of one's willingness to arrest hair growth through energy.

To what extent do you wish to achieve a smooth body?
- I want to but I don't really have time.
- I want to but I am not sure of the scientific spiritual method.
- I'm ready to do anything and will adopt the method.

Do you have time during the day to do the treatment?
- Plenty of time; talking to hair is my new hobby.
- I'm too busy to find time to relate to it properly.
- I need to think about it and make sure that I will find the required time.

Do you have any particular body part you would like to start with?
- Yes, the entire body at the same time.
- One body part in particular.
- A particular body part of my partner's.

Are you willing to try an energetic treatment on yourself?
- Only if there is a one hundred percent success rate.
- I'm allergic.
- I understand and I want to do it.

Do you believe in your ability to bring about a change in your body?
- It sounds logical.
- This is spiritual bullshit.
- I'm the boss.

Are you willing to do the treatment to inspire someone else?
- Of course, I'll be a pioneer for family and friends.
- I won't discuss how I succeeded.
- I don't know if I'll succeed.

How much time are you willing to invest daily in nurturing your body?
- The entire day.
- A little bit of time without effort.
- How would you define "nurturing?"

Can you imagine yourself with a smooth body?
- I don't know how to imagine things.
- Sure, I can see myself already really excited.
- If I make a great effort.

Who is responsible for removing hair from your body?
- The beautician.
- Me.
- My husband/mother pays for the treatments.

What do you tend to do in situations of uncertainty/discomfort?
- Carry on.
- Analyze the situation.
- Deal with it.

How do you usually react when encountering skeptical people?
- It makes me less confident in myself.
- I ignore them.
- I listen to myself.

When you achieve a smooth, hairless skin, what will you say to yourself?
- Not bad.
- Wow, rejoice!
- Damn, it works.

Tips

Don't tell anyone that you are energetically stopping the growth of your hair until you see results. Other peoples' doubts could lower your morale.

Our attitude to removing hair is usually negative, impatient, painful, frustrating and constricting. The energetic arrest of hair growth starts with changing our attitude towards hair and its presence on our body. We need to accept it compassionately and inclusively, with awareness and acceptance of the fact that hair exists and there is no point in fighting against it. All we can do is choose to change it.

Start the energy treatment knowing that you are a vessel of influence that can change the hair vibration within your body according to your wishes.

The words, imagination, and feeling of connection that I've found with hair are not the only way to cause hair to stop growing. You need to understand the energetic law of nature regarding hair. Trust what **feels** good to you, including your imagination and the emotion that flows easily within you.

When you understand the scientific logic of influencing hair, the rational mind can still distract you through reluctance to do the energetic treatment. This can happen repeatedly before a treatment. It is mostly related to forgetting about the existing reality of vibrations or the conscious transition to a wonderful, good intention. But once you are feeling the emotion, the process flows with ease.

Remember! Simply start. The process won't require many treatments if the quality of each treatment is deep and focused.

It isn't always easy to enjoy the **journey** of stopping the growth of hair when the desire for this process is great. This can hamper the joy in the process and also harm the speed of the results. This is why you should adopt a calm, joyful approach of satisfaction for the information and the acceleration of the process with each treatment.

Although each treatment is brief, we produce energy through emotion. You need focus, determination, and persistence, like any process. The hair will weaken during the process, but this will occur quickly enough to offer evidence of results.

There may be spot treatments when you feel more connected to emotion and the action of talking to hair and days when you feel disconnected and void of energy. It's okay. The important thing is to go on and persevere. When positive results are evident, the treatment will become easier, and your enthusiasm and belief will increase from the very recognition that your hair is responding to you and the treatment is working for you.

Emotion at Work

Writing focuses one's desire and intention, thereby reinforcing emotion.
Choose one body part and write down **why** you want the skin to be permanently smooth and hairless.

_____

_____

_____

_____

_____

_____

_____

How will you **feel** when the skin of this body part is permanently smooth and hairless?

I'd like to hear about your experience with energy hair removal treatments, including the images you used to visualize it, and the feeling that came about from the arrest of hair growth.

If you have any questions, please contact me:
ehair@gmail.com

Printed in Great Britain
by Amazon